SIX AGELESS PRINCIPLES FOR LONG LIFE SUCCESS

LIVE A LONGER HEALTHIER LIFE & APPEAR DECADES YOUNGER

ANDREW L. OLIVER

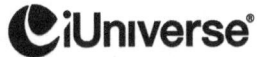

SIX AGELESS PRINCIPLES FOR LONG LIFE SUCCESS
LIVE A LONGER HEALTHIER LIFE & APPEAR DECADES YOUNGER

iUniverse books may be ordered through booksellers or by contacting:

iUniverse
1663 Liberty Drive
Bloomington, IN 47403
www.iuniverse.com
1-800-Authors (1-800-288-4677)

ISBN: 978-0-5952-1470-9 (sc)
ISBN: 978-1-4759-1716-1 (e)

Print information available on the last page.

iUniverse rev. date: 06/12/2019

CONTENTS

LIST OF ILLUSTRATIONS

To Juan Ponce de Leon

Who like many of us, searched for the fountain of youth outside himself; when all the time it was inside his body just waiting to be found.

ACKNOWLEDGEMENTS

This book could not have been written without the help and inspiration of many people who I know personally and vicariously.

Thank you Dad for being an inspiration to me as a father. You provided many insights that dramatically improved this book. Thank you Mom for all your love. Much of who I am is a reflection of the values you and Dad imparted to me.

Thank you Morris Landis for being a living example on how to live the principles of this book. Your wise counsel and your friendship has blessed my life. Thank you Derrick Whitfield, for all your kind words of encouragement when you saw the first draft. Your enthusiastic response encouraged me to continue.

Thank you Dr. Wayne Dyer for influencing my thoughts in so many ways. Thank you Les Brown Jr. for motivating me through the tough times. Thank you Jim Rohn for making self-help as easy to understand as an apple a day or a walk around the block. Thank you Patricia Fripp for advising me not to distribute this book if I needed to make excuses for it. Thank you Deepak Chopra for providing me with a vocabulary to describe mind and body communication at the cellular level. Thank you Louise Hay for helping me remove the word should from my vocabulary and from this book.

Thank you to Michelle Lubaczewski, Larry Dillon and Lee Oliver for helping with the editing of this book.

Thank you Pro Tim for the back cover photography and Steve and Pat Goodman for the book photography.

FOREWORD

You are encouraged to share the "secrets" in this book with those you love because it can be painful for all concerned if you don't. It may be painful for you to watch your friends and loved ones grow old and die before your eyes and before their time. It may be painful for them because they see themselves aging while you don't and burn with envy.

This book is not a study in mysticism, metaphysics, and the like; rather it is a practical approach to living a full and enriched life, with the face and body that belies your chronological age by ten, twenty, or more years. You can slow down the rate at which you age and live longer, and retain a youthful look, a zest for life, and the ability to do all the things that you want. Furthermore, you can maintain this youthful appearance and vitality well past what we now consider old age.

Ask yourself what is old age? What do you mean when you say you are reaching middle age, or growing old? Is it the proverbial "70 or 80 years" you believe is promised in the bible? Is it much more? Can you really live to ages of 120 years or more and still remain active, healthy, and lucid? The answer is "Yes you can." You have programmed yourself to believe that your lifetime must fit in a certain window--either because of heredity, environment, or some other known or unknown controlling factor that determines how long you live. When you learn that living a long and healthful life--well over a hundred years--is not only a possibility, but also a very high probability, you may make a commitment to changing your lifestyle and enhancing the factors that bring about this extension of your life cycle.

Believe that it is possible to live 120 years in excellent health

The Guinness Book of World Records lists Jeanne Louise Calment as the oldest person to ever live, for persons whose birth date could be authenticated by reliable records. She lived 122 years and 5 months. She was born on February 21, 1875 in Arles France and had become the greatest attraction to that city since the artist Vincent Van Gogh, who spent a year there in 1888. She met him that year when he came to her uncle's shop to buy paints, and later remembered him as *"dirty, badly dressed and disagreeable.[1]"* She died on August 4, 1997. Since she is the only person documented to live past 120 years, and there are about 6 billion people inhabiting planet earth, you could surmise that the odds of living that long are 6 billion to one. Not very good odds if you are a betting person.

Well, prior to May 6, 1954, no person had ever run the mile faster than 4 minutes. Before this date, medical science had all the biological complications, and physics had all the mathematical theories, as to why it was impossible. But all things are possible to those who believe. Roger Bannister believed and ran the mile in 3:59.4. Was science wrong? Of course not! It's just that the people using the science were biased in the observation of what was possible. Are the odds one in six billion that anyone else could do it since Bannister was the only one? To date, more than 700 runners have broken 4:00 minutes since Bannister opened our mind (source: Track & Field News July 1994).

Therefore, if Jean Louise Calment of France could live 120 years then so can you. Believe you can live 120 years in excellent health and then go about the task of making it a reality. If you believe you can or believe you cannot, you are probably right. Believe you can do it.

Scientific evidence proves 120 years is possible

One of the most respected scientists studying aging is Walter M. Bortz II M.D. He is former president of the American Geriatrics Society with over 35 years of clinical experience. He co-chaired the AMA-ANA Task

---

[1] Jeanne Calment, world's oldest person, dies at 122, Jocelyn Noveck, Associated Press, August 4, 1997.

Force on Aging, and is presently Clinical Associate Professor at Stanford University Medical School. He is the author of the highly acclaimed book, *We Live Too Short and Die Too Long.* In this book he states,

> "It is my best estimation that our biogenetic maximum life span is 120 years-approximately 1 million hours. This means that at birth we have the capacity to live that long--presuming that nothing happens to us in the meantime. The lines of evidence that lead to this conclusion are several, and while no single one can constitute definitive proof, taken together they achieve a high level of probability. Such reasoning is termed the Principle of Invariance.
>
> Using this principle, I find five lines of evidence to support my thesis (i.e. that your maximum life span is 120 years). These are: observational data, biostatistical maneuvers, the correlations between longevity and skeletal maturation, studies regarding the decline of vital organ function, and research into the longevity of cells in controlled environments."

The Bible says your life span is 120 years

Many people incorrectly believe the bible states that our life span is 70 to 80 years. The interpretation of scripture used to support this number is Psalm 90 verse 10.

> "Seventy years are given to us! Some may even reach eighty. But even the best of these years are filled with pain and trouble; soon they dissapear and we are gone."

This is the scripture that is read at a lot of funerals, it is somewhat appropriate. Statistically, the person in that casket is 80 years old or less and those last days were filled with pain.

Let's first put this scripture in the proper perspective. This was not God speaking to man, but man speaking to God. It was a prayer by

Moses, and in many ways he was complaining to God about the fact that many people were dying too young and in a weak state. He was asking God to give people the wisdom to correctly live their lives and increase their life span (Psalm 90:12).

The scripture in the bible where God tells mankind how long they can live is found in Genesis 6:3. It states,

> "Then the Lord said, "My Spirit will not put up with humans for such a long time for they are only mortal flesh, in the future they will live no more than 120 years."

And the 120 years referred to in the bible is not filled with age related disease and pain. It is 120 years of healthy vigor and vitality. Moses is the classic example of how the bible states you can live and ultimately die. Deuteronomy 34:5-7 states,

> "Moses was 120 years old when he died, yet his eyesight was clear and he was strong as ever."

Summary

There are no tricks to changing your habits, and consequently your daily actions, to enable you to appear decades younger, and live a longer healthier life. It only takes an awareness of how your everyday habits cause you to age in a manner that nature has not intended. There are several basic steps you must follow, and you will soon see and feel the results of your new commitment to living longer and healthier. The steps are identified here and are discussed in detail, along with how to implement them in subsequent chapters.

The six ageless principles for long life success are:
1. Relax your mind and body with spiritual recreation.
2. Cultivate positive healthy relationships and eliminate the negative.
3. Think and grow healthy, wealthy, and wise.
4. Invest more on yourself than you do on your job and possessions.

5. Exercise before eating and thoroughly flush your system.
6. Refuse to age gracefully.

You will find the above steps to be sound practices that can enable you to slow down the process of aging and restore to your body the vitality and looks of one considerably younger than present--regardless of how old you now are. This book provides a complete skill set that produces an ageless body that can live 120 years. These new skills exercise your mind, body and spirit. You are cautioned to take on one or two of these new skills at a time. Attempting to do everything at once might be too overwhelming. Master each skill until it becomes a habit, and then begin to acquire another. Learn them, practice them, teach them, and relish the remarkable results.

Relax your mind and body with spiritual recreation

Your quest for ageless long life must begin from the inside--and not from the outside. You have just begun a unique quest of aging slower and living longer by focusing first on the unseen part of your being, and then gradually moving towards the seen. Aging occurs because of stresses related to the following areas:

1. Energy
2. Thoughts
3. Attitudes
4. Feelings
5. Wear and tear on the internal organs and system of your body
6. Wear and tear on the external appearance of your body

The first four items are invisible. You cannot see energy, feelings, thoughts, or attitudes--you can only deal with the results they produce. Whereas, you can see the last two items on the list--namely, the effects of aging on your physical body. This is why most books and programs dealing with aging slower or living longer focus primarily on these visible areas. They relate the aging process to three areas: diet, nutrition and exercise. Thus, most people who are trying to live longer and age slower spend 100% of their time covering only 30 percent of the areas that will cause them to age slower, and neglect the remaining 70 percent because it intuitively does not appear to matter. But matter it does; the weight of the unseen weights heavily on the seen.

To illustrate how invisible stress affects the rate of aging, imagine that you will attempt to bench press one-and-a-half times your body weight. If you are a person who weighs 160lbs that means you will attempt to bench press 240 pounds. For an average person in excellent shape this is a realistic goal, but will require hard work to achieve. As you lift the weigh from the bar, you hold your breath; your arms shake under the stress and you gently lower the bar to your chest. Then with all your might, you strain as you lift the bar back up and place it on the rack. Invisible stress based on feeling, thoughts and attitudes are similar to lifting a heavy weight and carrying the load of heavy stress internally. This invisible stress ages you just as fast as poor habits of diet, nutrition, and exercise. Listed below are just a few of the situations where this invisible stress accelerates your aging:

- Your mind is constantly filled with the clutter of unhealthy thoughts.
- Your emotional energy is blocked because of past trauma.
- Your body does not receive enough oxygen due to poor breathing habits.
- You worry over unfulfilling relationships with family, friends and lovers.
- You constantly worry over how to make, keep, and spend money.
- You stress out over growing old in a culture that worships youth.

You will learn methods to relax, renew, and re-energize your spirit to provide you with the fresh perspective and energy necessary to live out your days to their full number. Many people are burning out spiritually. Stress, worry, and poor habits of living, all contribute to their early demise. You will learn physical exercises that build up the spiritual nature of your life. We call this spiritual nature your soul.

Almost any exercise can be transformed into a spiritual experience with a little thought. The exercises discussed in this chapter are tai chi, meditation, and yoga. Tai chi allows you to relax and find balance in all your movements. Meditation allows you to relax and enjoy the present moment. Yoga allows you to relax while your body becomes more flexible. While doing these exercises your mind is focused on a spiritual lesson. When exercise is combined with conscious breathing and spiritual lessons it transforms mere physical activity into a euphoric mind, body and spirit experience.

> **Theory: If people were candles, then many people die with plenty of wax remaining on the wick. They burn out. Live to your full potential and burn up all the wax.**

Candles are an excellent metaphor of human life. The candle wax and wick represents your potential and physical nature. The candle flame represents your spiritual nature. Without the flame the candle is useless. Yet, there is a fragile link between life and death, between the candle's flame shining brightly and suddenly being extinguished. You are born into the world with a set amount of time to exist--a certain amount of wax. Spiritual relaxation exercises strengthen your flame and allow you to burn up all the wax of your life span candle.

Since most people die early, we have mistakenly assumed that the candle life span is only 80 years at best. We feel that if a person lives to the age of 80, that their life was long and their days were many. Yet the reality is there could have been another 40 years of healthy living, if their candlestick was better maintained or their flame was better protected.

Understanding how spiritual energy increases life span

The source of all energy for humans comes from light. Light is absorbed by green plants in a process called photosynthesis and produces the oxygen you breathe. As the plants grow they are eaten and serve as the first part of your food chain. The food is digested and metabolized by your body and your energy is produced in cells called mitochondria. The mitochondria produce energy in the body in a substance called ATP (adenosine triphosphate). This energy flows throughout your body and is used to fuel your physical efforts. The word calorie describes how the body burns ATP as fuel.

Energy also has a spiritual nature that was eloquently described by Dr. Albert Einstein, when he said, *"Energy is never created or destroyed; it only transfers into another form."* This is important to you since your source of life is your energy. Therefore you must look at ways to keep that energy circulating in your healthy body for as long as possible.

Breathe deeply and slowly to energize your cardiovascular system

In the same way that oxygen when added to fire increases the flame, increasing the oxygen to your body increases your vitality and awareness. Large doses of oxygen on a daily basis are necessary for high energy. Aerobic exercise provides a means to increase your breathing by exerting your muscles to oxygen depletion. You can garner many of the same benefits of exercising without all the physical effort simply by breathing deeply and slowly every day.

Stop for a moment and notice how you are breathing right now. The average person takes about 18-20 breaths in a minute and these breaths are short and shallow. In essence you are only utilizing half of your lung capacity with each breath. Scientists have already proven that humans only utilize a small portion of their brain's capacity. Likewise, you are only using a small portion of your lung's capacity.

Take 10 minutes each day breathing in deep and slow breaths, filling your lungs all the way and then exhaling very slowly. Your breaths will be so deep and slow that it takes you 10 seconds to inhale and 6 seconds to exhale, thereby reducing your breaths per minute from 18 to about 5. Do this for 3 minutes at first till you can reach around 10 minutes straight. When doing this exercise inhale through your nose and exhale through your mouth. This exercise vitalizes your body with massive doses of oxygen, and gives you a natural high from the oxygen for several hours. Try to do this exercise 3 times per day.

Meditate to energize your mind and nerveous system

Meditation is a technique to quiet your mind and allows you to hear from the wisdom of the universe. The endless chatter of your mental self-talk becomes tiresome to your mind and body. You are constantly talking to yourself all the time. And clearly, if you are always talking then you never get to hear what the universal intelligence has to say. It drains your mental energy in stress and blocks the creative ideas that can inspire you to higher levels of living.

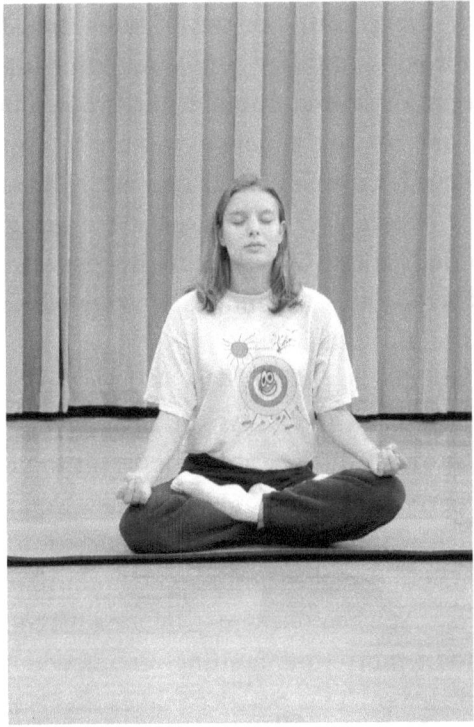

Figure 1—Full Lotus Meditation Position

Tich Nat Hahn, a Vietnamese Buddhist monk who was nominated by Dr. Martin Luther King Jr. for the Nobel Peace prize, developed mindfulness meditation. Mindfulness meditation is powerful because it blends the power of silence with mindful breathing, visualization, and positive affirmation to create a present moment experience that relaxes the mind, body, and spirit. This meditation has 5 key exercises with an affirmation that is accompanied by a visualization to provide a specific benefit. Each affirmation is merged with a specific visualization to create a powerful effect on your mind, body and spirit. The exercises are: in/out, flower/fresh, mountain/solid, water/reflecting and space/free.

The first and core aspect of Mindfulness meditation is **in/out** which is mindful breathing. The benefit it provides is to merge your mind and body and keep you in the present moment. First, find a quiet place to sit and close your eyes. Then breathe in deeply and slowly and as you breathe in, think or say, **"I know that I am breathing in."** Feel the air enter your lungs and circulate throughout your body. Then as you exhale slowly and evenly, think or say, **"I know that I am breathing out."** Feel the air leaving your body and circulating in the atmosphere. Repeat this process for several minutes until your thoughts and your actions become one. At this moment you are totally in the present moment. Your focus is on who you are and what you are doing, which is breathing. Few people ever truly experience being in the present moment. Their minds always take them to the past or to the future. The present moment is the only time and place where relaxation, creativity, and infinite possibilities can occur.

The second exercise is **flower/fresh**. When you breathe in, think or say, **"I see myself as a flower."** As you breathe out, think or say, **"I feel fresh."** With this meditation it is important to visual yourself as a flower or see in your mind a flower. Visualize yourself sitting on a lotus flower. When you breathe out it is important to smile. Smiling releases endorphins and makes you happy. Endorphins are powerful neurotransmitters that when released produce a narcotic and euphoric effect stronger than morphine. Smiling also makes the people that receive your smile happy. This practice makes every cell in your body smile like a flower and become fresh again. You become fresh again for yourself and all those around you. This meditation is a good way to refresh yourself so that you and all around you are at peace. Otherwise, when you have too many worries and anger, you are not sitting on a lotus flower, you are sitting on hot coals and you have no peace.

The third exercise is called **mountain/solid**. When you breathe in, think or say, **"I see myself as a mountain,"** as you exhale, think or say, **"I feel solid."** This exercise brings stability to the body first by being grounded in a full or half lotus meditation position. In this position you are strong and solid and you must visualize yourself as a mountain. In essence you become solid in both body and mind. Many times strong emotions such as anger, despair or fear overwhelm you and if you are not trained on how to handle your emotions, you suffer so much and may even take your own life. That is why this meditation is so important. It teaches that you are grounded and are more solid than your emotions. That is why you must practice this exercise everyday so that when powerful emotions occur you will have the strength to handle them. This meditation may someday save your life.

The fourth exercise is **water/reflecting**. In this meditation you must visualize a pond where the water is so still and clear that it reflects without distortion the mountains and the blue sky. If you took a picture of the pond, your reflection is crystal clear. As you breathe in, think or say, **"I see myself as still waters."** As you breathe out, think or say, **"I reflect things as they are."** When you are calm you receive the truth from other people without distortion. If the water of your pond is not calm everything you see becomes distorted and therefore it is not the fault of what others do that makes for your unhappiness, it is the distortion in the pond of your mind that is causing your unhappiness. If your perceptions are clear then you hear the truth that the cosmos tries to tell you and have true understanding and happiness.

The fifth exercise is **space/free**. Breathing in, think or say, **"I see myself as space."** Breathing out, think or say **"I feel free."** Space is the symbol of liberty. Without enough space you may not be happy. If you have so many projects and worries there is no space for you to enjoy happiness. Therefore you must have space inside and outside of yourself to be truly happy. If you want your lover to be happy give him or her some space. Otherwise, you cramp their liberty and they feel unhappy. Practicing this meditation improves the quality of your relationships.

Practice Kundalini yoga to energize your endocrine system

Just like your body has a system to circulate blood, oxygen, food, and sensory perception, it also has a system to circulate energy. A description of this system comes from the Indian yogis and is called the chakra energy system. Chakra is a Sanskrit word, which means a wheel, or disc or any arrangement in a circular form.

The chakra system contains seven locations throughout the body. Each location is linked to a gland in the endocrine system. Together with the nervous system and various hormones secretions, the chakras enable you to react to changes in your environment, both internal and external. Each chakra location provides a physical benefit and a spiritual metaphor.

Kundalini yoga exercises stimulate the energy flow through the chakra system. Kundalini is a Sanskrit word that means spiral or coiled power. It is like a serpent that lies coiled while sleeping. It combines movement, imagery and breathing to stimulate the nerves and endocrine glands to unblock the chakra centers and keep the energy flowing throughout your body.

Exercise the first chakra to control your fear and anger

The first chakra is located at the base of your spine. It is physically connected with your adrenal glands. The adrenal glands produce adrenalin necessary to fight or flee danger. When this hormone is out of balance your body does not metabolize water and salt efficiently and you can become over anxious. The spiritual metaphor of this chakra is related to your need to survive and prosper in relationship to your basic needs. Like Maslow's hierarchy of needs this is the lowest level of living and yet the most necessary. When this chakra is out of balance it is manifest in excess worry and unnecessary strife. You know this chakra is out of balance by overwhelming feelings of need, which is manifested negatively as greed. There are only six things your body needs for the pursuit of life and liberty:

- Light--necessary for sight and the ability for plant life to grow
- Nutritious food--necessary for the sustenance of the body
- Pure and fresh water--necessary for the sustenance of the body
- Shelter--necessary to protect the body from the elements
- Air--necessary to supply the cells with oxygen
- Love--necessary to give life meaning and purpose

In addition to these physical needs, in the audio program *Personal Power II: The Driving Force*, Anthony Robins documents 6 human needs for the pursuit of happiness. These needs are:

- Certainty--to know that some things in life are stable and not chaotic

- Uncertainty--to make life exciting and not repetitively mundane
- Significance--to know that your life is important
- Connection--to belong to a group and not feel alone
- Growth--to know that you can become more than you already are
- Contribution--to give back some of what you have received

Outside of these needs everything else is just a want and not a need. The element that rules this chakra is earth. Earthly relates to being grounded in the things of this world, as in the sense of worldly versus spiritual.

Exercises to do for the first chakra are chants, **Breath-of-fire breathing**, Spine Flexors and Frog Pose. The chant is *Ong Namo Guru Dev Namo*. This chant translates to *"I bow to the infinite energy within myself."* Breath-of-fire breathing stimulates the energy flow through your body. This breath is shallow and rapid, inhaling and exhaling through your nose.

To do frog pose you need to get in the position where you would jump like a frog. Stand up and then crouches down with knees bent, until your buttocks touch the back of your calves. Then place your hands between your legs and touch the ground with the palms of your hands. This is frog position. Slowly raise your hips until your legs are as straight as possible without removing your hands from the ground. While moving the hips up, lower the head so that it is hanging downward. Then slowly bend your knees again, raising your head so that when you are fully crouched, you are looking straight ahead. Do this movement while doing the **breath-of-fire breathing**.

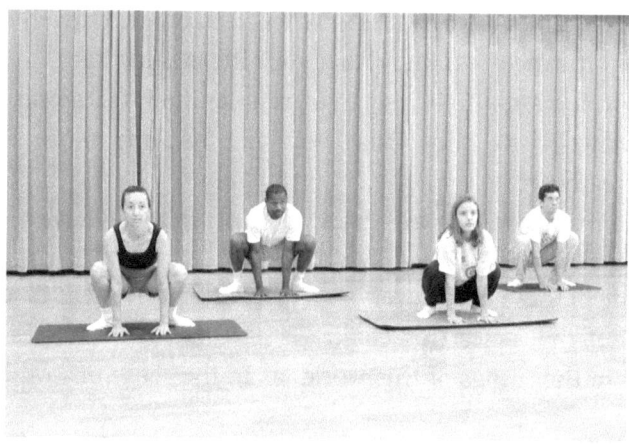

Figure 2—Starting Position for Frog Pose

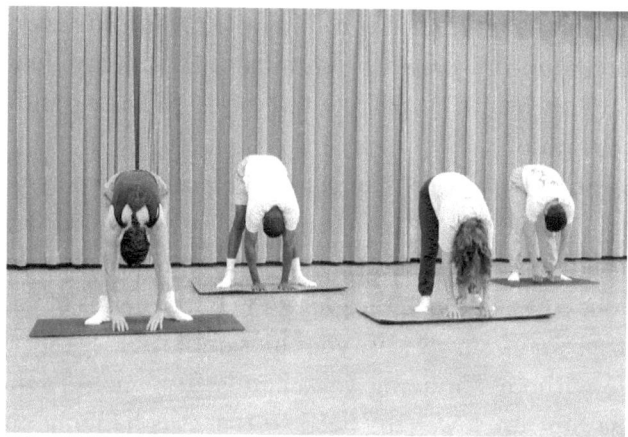

Figure 3—Ending Position for Frog Pose

Spine Flexors start in seated yoga position with your hands on your knees, and then flex your head back while you flex your spine in toward your stomach. Then flex your head forward, placing your chin on your chest, while you flex your spine out toward your back. When done correctly, your spine should mimic the movements of a snake moving up a wall. Do this movement while doing the **breath-of-fire breathing**. Repeat these movements for 3 to 5 minutes. As you do these exercises visualize your energy shining like a beam of light into the universe from your first chakra.

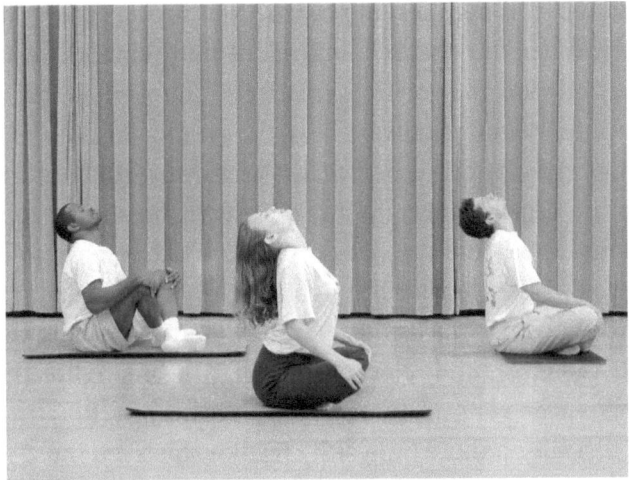

Figure 4—Starting position for Spine Flexors

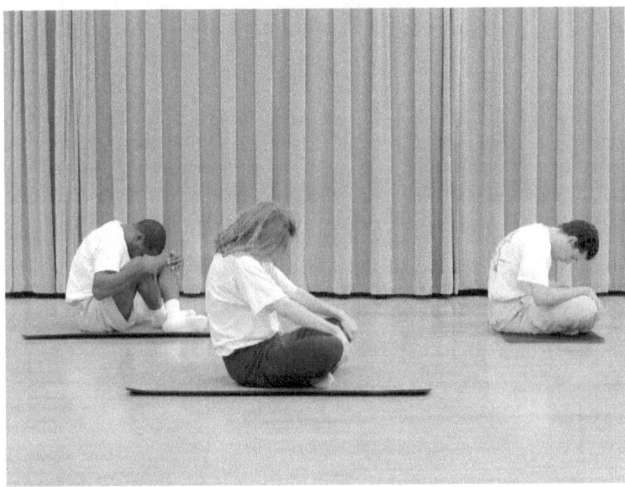

Figure 5—Ending position for Spine Flexors

Exercise the second chakra to improve your romance and creativity

The second chakra is located within your sexual organs. It is physically connected with your gonads or ovaries. These glands produce testosterone in men or estrogen and progesterone in women. When these hormones are out of balance your body may have difficult reproducing offspring. The spiritual metaphor of this chakra is related to your need to be creative and produce what you need to survive. When this chakra is out of balance it is manifest in promiscuous sexual activity or a block in creativity. When this chakra is in balance your romantic relationships are healthy and vital and you flow creatively. The element that rules this chakra is water. Water has always been the symbol for life and creation.

Exercises to do for the second chakra are **Oh-breath** breathing, Pelvic Rotations and Hip Openers. With **Oh-breath** breathing you breathe through your mouth and you pucker your lips like you are going to kiss someone. You will also exhale through your mouth. Pelvic rotations start in seated yoga position with your hands on your knees, and then rotate your pelvis and upper body clock wise doing **Oh-breath** breathing. This exercise focuses on your relationships that are healthy. Rotating counter clockwise focuses on those unhealthy relationships you must set free.

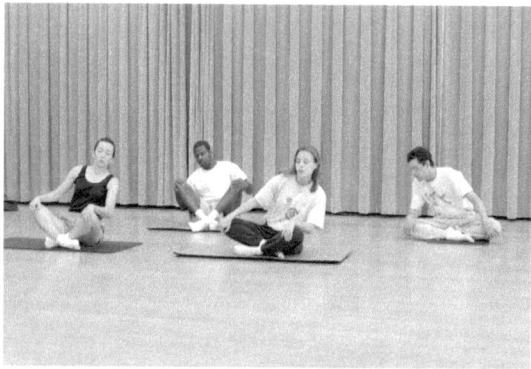

*Figure 6—Pelvic Rotations to the right to
strengthen relationships and creativity*

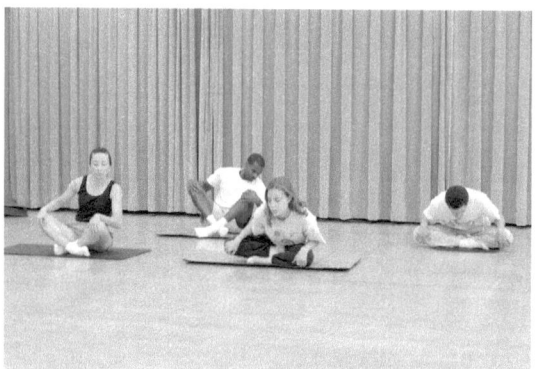

*Figure 7—Pelvic Rotations to the left release
unhealthy relationships and creativity blocks*

To do hip openers lay on your back with your hands at your side. Bring your legs and knees up to your chest and then spread them so they form the letter "V." With each breath rotate the legs to one side and bring in one leg, and when rotating to the other side, bring in that leg while extending the other. As you do these exercises visualize your energy shining like a beam of light into the universe from your second chakra.

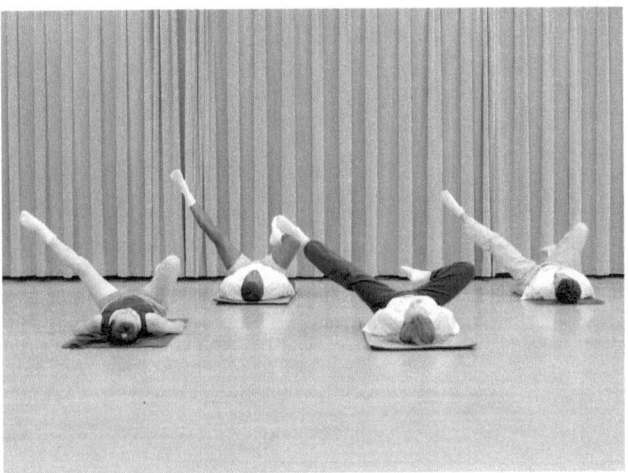

Figure 8—Starting position for Hip Openers on the inhale

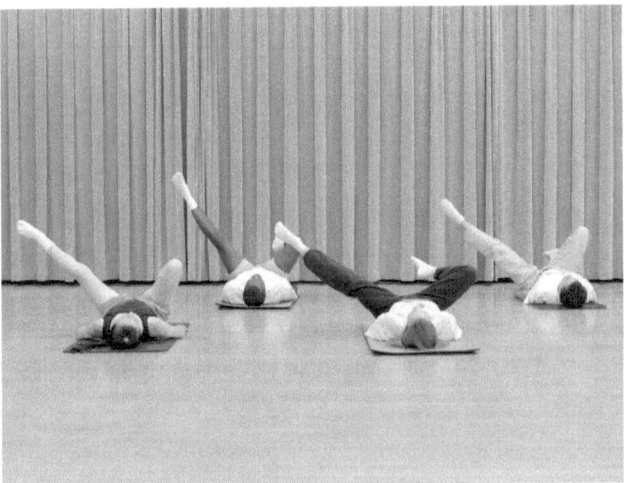

Figure 9—Starting position for Hip Openers on the exhale

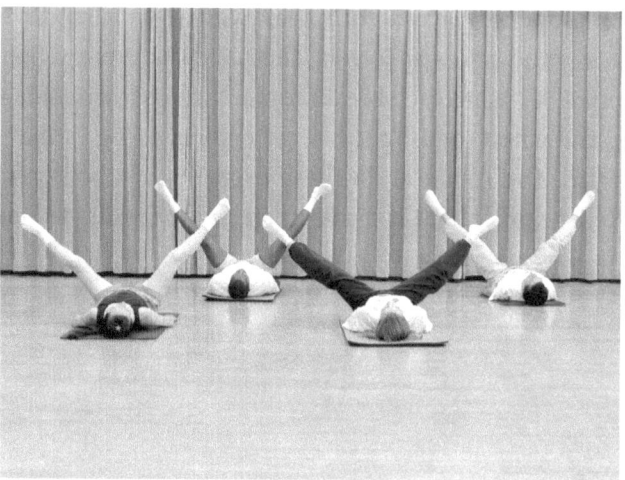

Figure 10—Ending position after doing a set of Hip Openers

Exercise the third chakra to control your need for power over others

The third chakra is located within your stomach area. It is physically connected with your pancreas. These glands produce insulin and glycogen. When this hormone is out of balance blood sugar levels in your body are affected and diabetes could result. The spiritual metaphor of this chakra is related to your need for personal power. When this chakra is out of balance you feel powerless in your work relationships or you may act like an egomaniac. When this chakra is in balance you feel strong and in control without being overbearing. The element that rules this chakra is fire. Fire represents the "burning" desire as fire in the belly.

Exercises to do for the third chakra are the Pelvic Arch and Stretch pose. To do the Pelvic Arch exercise, lie on your back. Then bend your knees and place your feet close to your hips. Take your arms and point them up towards the sky. Connect the fingertips from both hands forming a steeple over your heart. As you inhale, slowly lower your arms above your head with the arms still connected as a steeple over your head when your arms are on the ground. As you lower the arms, pretend a string is attached to your navel and lifts your stomach as you arch your back. As you exhale slowly raise your arms back above your heart and lower your stomach to the ground.

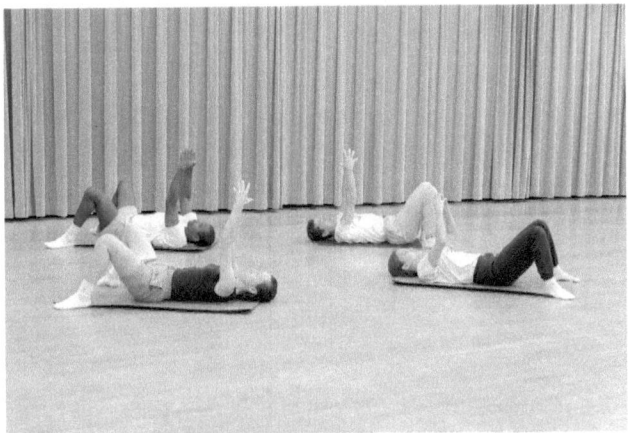

Figure 11—Starting position for Pelvic Arch Pose

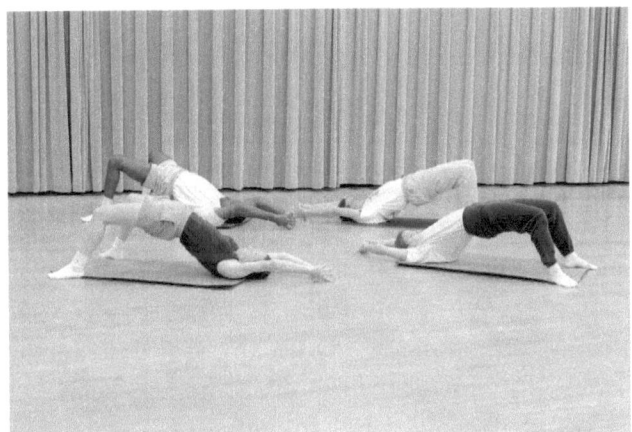

Figure 12—Ending position for Pelvic Arch Pose

Stretch pose requires you to lie on your back with your arms at your side. Then raise your feet off the ground 6 inches and point your toes. Lift your head and look out over your toes. In this position do **breath-of-fire** breathing. This is a difficult exercise to do. If you feel too much stress in your lower back then place your hands underneath your hips. In the beginning try to do this exercise 3 times for about 15 seconds each set. As your strength increases increase the duration to 3 minutes maximum. As you do these exercises visualize your energy shining like a beam of light into the universe from your third chakra.

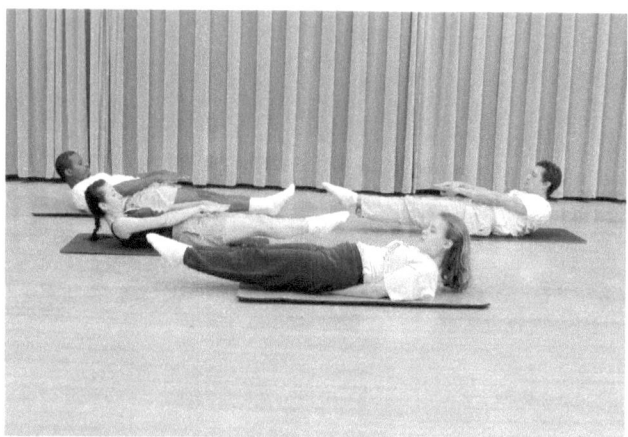

Figure 13—Stretch Pose with Breath-of-Fire breathing.

Exercise the fourth chakra to improve your friendships

The fourth chakra is located within your heart area. It is physically connected with your thymus glands. These glands aid in the production of white blood cells, which fight infection and disease. When this hormone is out of balance your resistance to sickness is lowered. The spiritual metaphor of this chakra is related to your need for platonic love and friendship. When this chakra is out of balance you feel your relationships are stressful. This is usually manifest during holiday seasons when you get physically sick due to holiday depression. When this chakra is in balance you feel strong and connected with family and friends. The element that rules this chakra is air. Air represents the symbiosis of all living things. Humans breathe oxygen and exhale carbon dioxide. Plants inhale carbon dioxide and exhale oxygen. This interaction sustains all life on the planet.

Exercises to do for the fourth chakra are Camel pose and **Who-Lah** breathing with Heart Opener pose. To do the Camel Pose, first sit on you knees and bend your back so that you can grab your ankles with your hands. If you cannot grab your ankles then grab your thighs. If you cannot grab your thighs then grab your hips. Once in this position, stick your chest out and drop your head back so that your neck is fully opened and rest in this position for about 30 seconds to one minute. From this position you will bend your back and drop down into wisdom pose. Repeat these movements for 3 to 5 minutes. Breathe normally as you repeat this movement

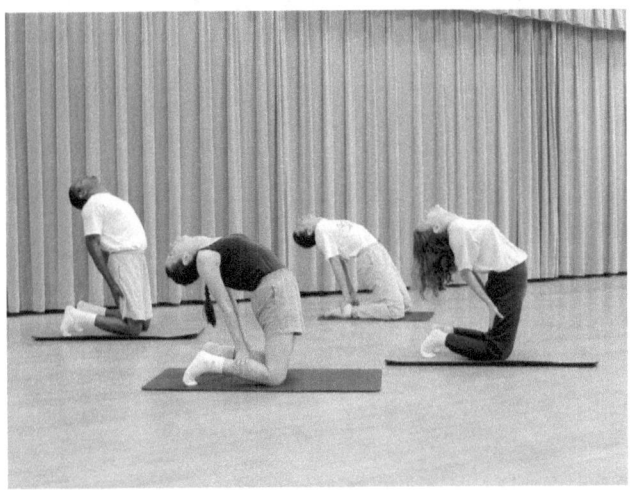

Figure 14—Starting position for Camel Pose

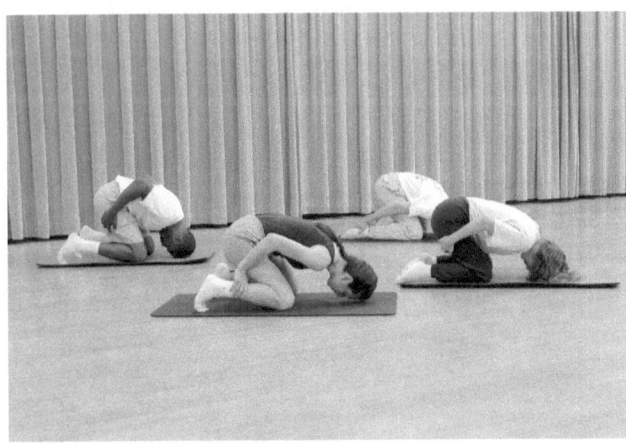

Figure 15—Ending position for Camel Pose

To do **Who-Lah** breathing, first take a large inhale through your mouth and make a **"Who"** sound by rounding the lips. The slowly exhale through your mouth making a **"Lah"** sound with your tongue. To do the heart opener exercises sit on your knees with your hips resting on the back of your feet. Place your hands in prayer position in front of your heart. As you inhale making the **Who** sound, spread your arms wide like bird wings, rise your hips and slowly raise your chest and arch back as far as possible feeling the chest area open up as you relax the neck and let the head drop. Then as you exhale with the **Lah** sound slowly go back to the original position. As you do these exercises visualize your energy shining like a beam of light into the universe from your fourth chakra.

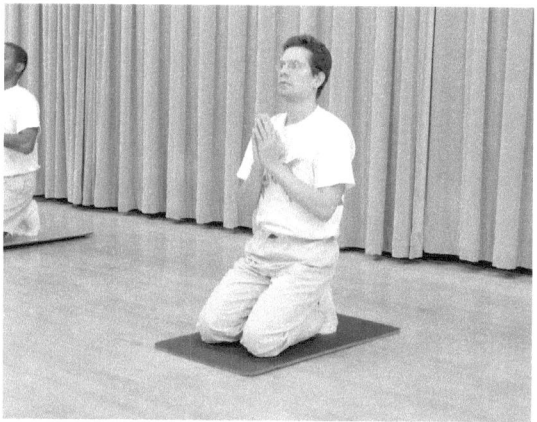

Figure 16—Begin the Heart Opener in Prayer Pose and as you move up make the Who sound.

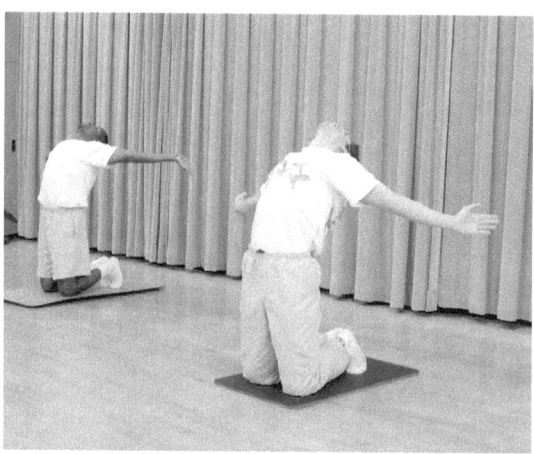

Figure 17—End Heart Openers by making the Lah sound as you go back to Prayer Pose

Exercise the fifth chakra to improve your communications

The fifth chakra is located within your throat area. It is physically connected with your thyroid glands. These glands secrete the hormone thyroxin, which controls the metabolism of food. When this hormone is out of balance your body may gain excessive weight, and you may have mood swings of depression. The spiritual metaphor of this chakra is related to communication. When this chakra is out of balance you feel like you are not being heard or understood clearly. When this chakra is in balance you feel connected when you communicate. The element that rules this chakra is ether. Ether represents the matter on which all communications travel. It is the portal to the spiritual realm of your universe. You cannot see radio waves or television waves, yet you know they travel on ether just like the sound of your voice does.

The exercise to do for the fifth chakra is **Satili** breathing with Cobra pose and **Wahe Guru** breathing with the Throat Opener pose. Cobra pose begins in wisdom pose. In this position you are sitting on your knees with your forehead on the floor and your arms extended in front of you. From Wisdom pose you will transfer your body to Cobra pose by extending your hips to the ground and arching the head back to stretch the chest. As you transition to Cobra pose you will begin **Satali** (pronounced Sit-ta-lee). **Satali** breathing is done by sticking your tongue out of your mouth and trying to form a loop from the center with your tongue. Then you will slowly inhale and exhale through your mouth. The exposed tongue cools the air as it enters your mouth. Once you are fully extended into Cobra pose you will go back to Wisdom pose. Repeat these movements for 3 to 5 minutes.

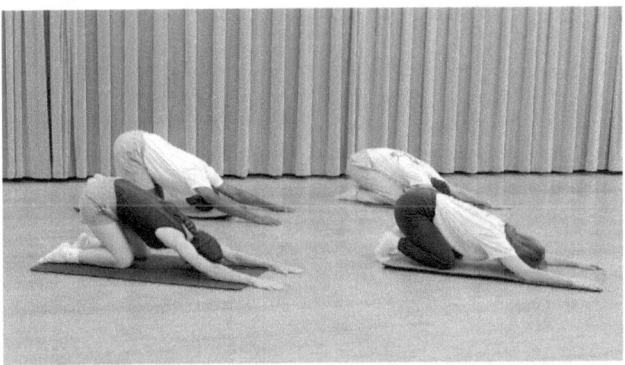

Figure 18—Starting position for Cobra Pose is Wisdom Pose

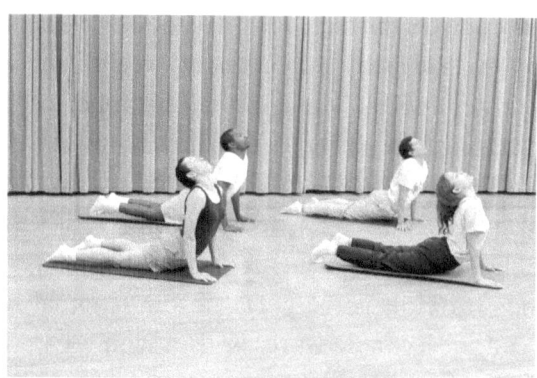

Figure 19—Ending position for Cobra Pose with Satili breathing

The exercise to do for the fifth chakra is **Wahe Guru** breathing with the Throat Opener pose. The sound **Wahe** means joy and ecstasy. The sound **Guru** means wisdom. This is the sound we make while breathing and doing the Throat Opener exercise. To do this exercise, stand and look straight ahead. Place your hands on your thigh and bend your knees so that you are in a comfortable position. Move your head so that you look over your right shoulder and make the sound **Wahe**. Then move you head so you look over your left shoulder and make the sound **Guru**. Repeat these movements for 3 to 5 minutes. As you rotate the neck and head, feel the throat muscle relax and stretch. As you do these exercises visualize your energy shining like a beam of light into the universe from your fifth chakra.

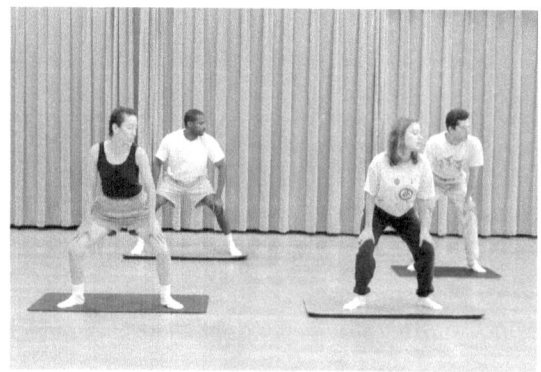

Figure 20—Say "Wahe" as you stretch
your neck and head to the right.

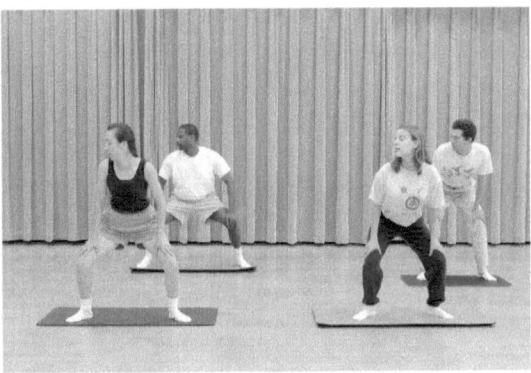

*Figure 21—Say "Guru" as you stretch
your neck and head to the left.*

Exercise the sixth chakra to improve your intution

The sixth chakra is located between your eyebrows in the location known as "the third eye." It is physically connected with your pineal gland. This gland affects the functions of the thyroid gland and the adrenal gland and gonads to control the onset of puberty. The spiritual metaphor of this chakra is related to your intuition. When this chakra is out of balance you don't listen or trust your intuitive feelings. When this chakra is in balance your intuition is strong and accurate. There are no elements that control this chakra because it is in the realm of the spiritual, which does not have known elements. The third eye is the portal that projects your thoughts from the physical dimension of your perceptions into the spiritual dimension of endless possibilities.

The exercise to do for the sixth chakra is Crow pose. The position for Crow starts similar to Frog Pose. Squat with you hands between your legs and you palms pressed against the ground. In this position you bow so that your third eye makes contact with the ground. As you lower your head to bow, press your elbows into yours legs to gain support. The grounding of your third eye represents that you trust your intuition to guide you in your earthly matters. Then rise up and go back to the original position. As you do these exercises visualize your energy shining like a beam of light into the universe from your sixth chakra.

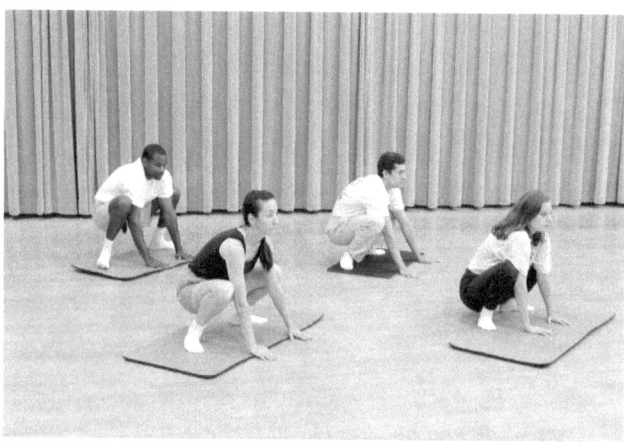

Figure 22—Starting position for Crow Pose

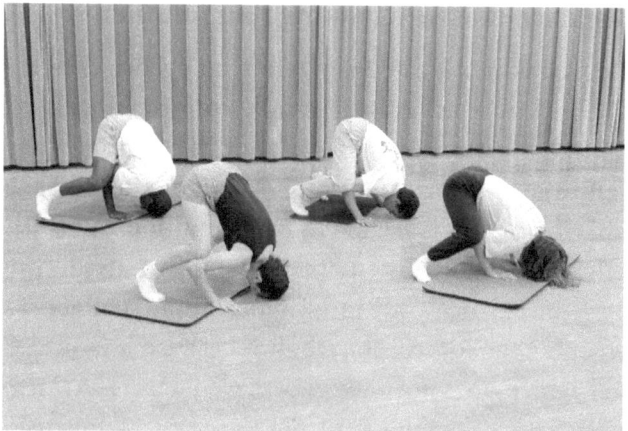

Figure 23—Ending position for Crow Pose

Exercise the seventh chakra to improve your spiritual awarness

The seventh chakra is located at the crown of your head. It is physically connected with your pituitary gland. This gland controls the functions of all the other glands. The spiritual metaphor of this chakra is related to your spirit nature. When this chakra is out of balance you don't feel connected spiritually. When this chakra is in balance you know that you and the creator are one. There are no elements that control this chakra because it is in the realm of the spiritual, which does not have known elements.

The exercise to do for the seventh chakra is Sphinx pose and **Sat Nam** pose. Sphinx pose starts in seated yoga position with your hands above the crown of your head with fingers interlaced. As you inhale you move your head back and your arms forward. As you exhale you move your head forward and your neck back. Think of this movement as polishing your halo or your aura. As you do this movement, close your eyes and look up with your eyes as if you were trying to see out of the crown of your head. Repeat these movements for 3 to 5 minutes.

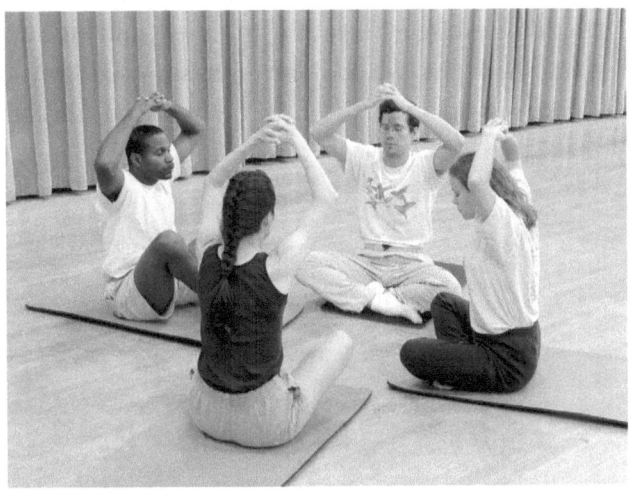

Figure 24—Starting position for Sphinx Pose

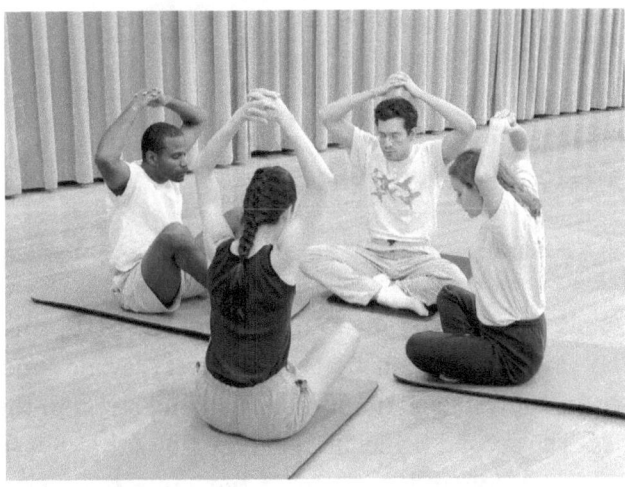

Figure 25—Ending position for Sphinx Pose

Sat Nam pose is done by sitting on your knees with your hands raised above your head connected and forming a steeple above the crown of your head. It is said that the crown of your head is the soft part of your skull where the soul enters during birth and where it departs when you expire. This exercise stimulates the crown chakra. As you inhale say the word **Sat** (which means Truth) and move your steeple towards the back of your head, while you move your head forward. Then as you exhale, say the word **Nam** (which means your name) and move your steeple towards the front of your head, while you move your head back. Do this exercise with your eyes closed, and look up through the crown of your head. As you do these exercises visualize your energy shining like a beam of light into the universe from your seventh chakra.

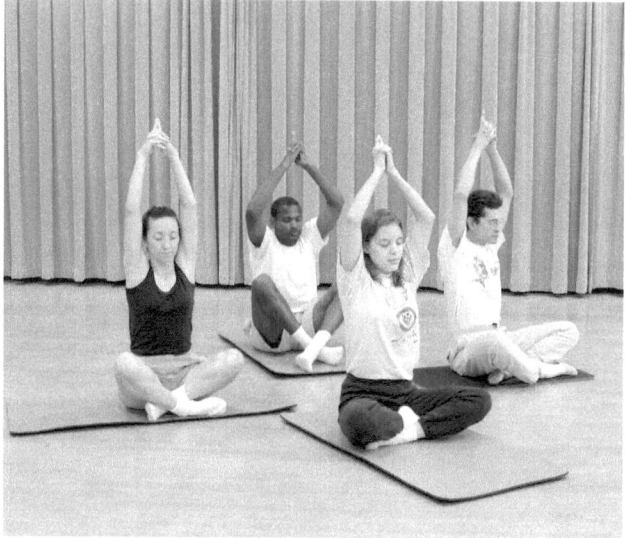

Figure 26—Sat Nam Pose

Practice Tai Chi to energize your musculosketal system

Tai Chi exercises are based on two principles. The first principle is to learn to relax your muscles and joints during everyday movement. Some people have an enormous amount of tension and stress in their joints and muscles. The second principle is energy flows through the joints; therefore when tension and stress are in the joints, the flow of energy is blocked. This blockage results in poor posture, high blood pressure, headaches, and sorted illness.

The goal of tai chi is to move slower, more relaxed, with deep breathing and focused concentration. Tai Chi is moving meditation. To the casual observer tai chi exercise is an enigma. How can an exercise that is so slow and relaxed provide any useful benefits to the body? When done correctly, tai chi allows your mind to merge and become one with your body. In this fast paced world of fight and flight, tai chi provides an alternative workout for the spirit. Tai Chi provides an exercise for those evolved beings that want to experience higher levels of consciousness.

Tai Chi has many health benefits. First it relieves stress in the bones and muscles that promote good posture. It benefits the muscles by working the opposite sides. Slow movements require endurance and therefore manipulate different muscle fibers in the body. Regular tai chi exercises allow your body to handle more stress. By providing for a full range of motion at a slow pace it allows the ligaments and cartilages to expand and contract to their full range of motion.

Let's perform a simple tai chi exercise to improve your posture and body alignment. The spiritual lesson of this exercise is that in life, you must walk upright before your fellow human beings and your spiritual creator. Being in alignment means that your thoughts, words and deeds are consistent and for the better good of those who come into contact with you. By placing your body into perfect alignment, you can instantly transform the moment into a spiritual experience just by the simple act of standing with good posture and remembering your spiritual lesson. Thus, standing erect transforms you into a spiritual experience while doing the most mundane tasks such as waiting in line or riding mass transit.

Find a wall with a flat surface you can stand against. Place the back of your head, your shoulder blades, your buttocks, and your heels against the wall. Your head must be in a position where your chin is parallel to the ground, and your eyes are looking straight ahead. Close your eyes and slowly move your arms from your side of your body to the top of your head as if you were doing jumping jacks with your arms only. Then bring your arms back down to your side. Practice this movement several times and each time moving the arms progressively slower. Try to think only of your movements. Once you can do this against the wall take one step away from the wall with your hand against your side and feel how perfect alignment feels. This might feel strange and unnatural and yet, it is absolutely the best posture you can have.

Listen only to the internal sounds of your body. As you slow down the pace you may notice that you hear your heart beat, feel the blood circulating through your veins, hear your nerve cells transmitting electrical energy. At this point your mind and body have become one. You may also notice that by doing this simple exercise for only 5 minutes, your arms may feel tired and you may want to rest. This is the beginning of a wonderful journey into the world of tai chi exercises. Every time you force your body into this posture and think on the spiritual lesson of alignment you are one with your mind, body, and spirit. The bibliography at the end of this chapter lists many good books and videotapes on tai chi.

Get the proper amounts of sleep to recharge your energy

Getting the proper amount of sleep is necessary to live a long and healthy life. You spend 1/3 of your existence in the state of sleep. Sleeping also provides a window into the afterlife and your true spiritual essence. Your spirit experiences conscious existence during waking hours and is limited by the physical laws of this universe. Whereas, when you sleep, your world is no longer limited. The world you experience during sleep is just as real as the world you experience while awake. The only difference is they are in two different dimensions. The former is in the dimension of the physical and the latter is in the dimension of endless possibilities. The Chinese philosopher Zhuangzi Chuang-tse (c.286 BCE) in the following story eloquently explains this difference.

> "Once Zhuang Zhou dreamed he was a butterfly, a fluttering butterfly. What fun he had, doing as he pleased! He did not know he was Zhou. Suddenly he woke up and found himself to be Zhou. He did not know whether Zhou had dreamed he was a butterfly or

a butterfly had dreamed he was Zhou. Between Zhou
and the butterfly there must be some distinction. This
is what is meant by the transformation of things."[2]

The trick to a truly happy life is to learn how to live while awake
in the dimension of endless possibilities. In order to do this you must
consistently get the proper amount of sleep under ideal circumstances.
Only you can determine the amount of sleep you need. This amount
of sleep is supported by your health and appearance. In other words,
you may get by consistently with only 4 hours of sleep but if you look
haggard and your thinking quickness is questionable, then 4 hours of
sleep is not good for you no matter how much money you're making.

To determine the amount of sleep you need practice without an
alarm clock over a long weekend. Go to bed at your normal time on a
Friday (assuming you don't work on weekends). Pretend you have to
work the next day and go through your usual routine during a workweek
night. But don't set an alarm clock, and see what time you arise the next
day. You will probably arise at the same time you usually do or within
30 minutes more or less. The reason this happens is your body is trained
to wake at a certain time. If you sleep more than one hour beyond your
normal waking time, then this is a clear indication that you are not
getting enough sleep. Continue the same experiment on Saturday and
Sunday night. Once you get a feel for the amount of sleep you need to
feel fully refreshed and awake, adjust the time you go to bed accordingly.

Try your best to go to bed at the same time and awake at the same
time every day of the week. Your sleep cycle works in a regular orbit
and requires consistency. Different sleeping habits on the weekend will
disrupt your cycle and prohibit your ability to ever get a consistent sleep
pattern.

Also, it is important that you don't eat at least 2 hours before you
go to sleep. When you sleep your body goes into repair mode. You don't
want your body to work on digestion during sleep since that decreases
the effectiveness of your sleep. Another good practice is to drink a glass
of water 2 hours before you go to sleep. This helps your body when it

---

[2] From Patricia Ebrey, Chinese Civilization: A Sourcebook, 2d ed. (New York:
Free Press, 1993), pp. 29

repairs itself during the sleep cycle. Many of the physical repairs need water. Drinking water 2 hours before going to sleep allows you to use the bathroom prior to going to bed and eliminates the urge to wake in the middle of the night to urinate.

Chanting, meditating, positive self-talk and prayer before you go to sleep is important to link the dimension of waking consciousness with the dimension of endless possibilities. Programming your conscious thoughts with the reality and results you desire before you go to sleep, influences the direction of your thoughts when you are in dream consciousness. In the dream consciousness you begin to act out the realities you desire and many time see the answers to achieving your goals. But the true power of this method is that your thoughts expand. The more time you spend seeing yourself doing and being the person you want, the easier it becomes to manifest this reality in waking consciousness.

Bibliography for the 1st Principle

1. 101 Essential Teps Basic Meditation, Naomi Ozaniec, DK Publishing, Inc
2. Alan Watts Teaches Meditation, Alan Watts, Audio Renaissance
3. Chakras Energy Centers of Transformation, Harish Johari, Destiny Books
4. Chakra Yoga, Gurutej Kaur, Sounds True Video
5. David Carradine's Tai Chi Workout, David Carradine, Goldhil Video
6. Fundamentals Tai Chi Fitness & Health, Joshua Grant, Video Treasures Inc.
7. Healing Reiki, Eleanor McKenzie, Ulysses Press
8. Kundalini Yoga The Flow of Eternal Power, Shakti Parwha Kaur Khalsa, Perigee Press
9. Kundalini Yoga with Gurmukh, Gurmkh, Livingarts
10. Personal Power II: The Driving Force, Anthony Robins, Nightingale Conant Co
11. Step-by-Step Tai Chi, Master Ham Kam Chuen, Simon & Schuster

12. The Art of Mindful Living, Thich Nhat Hanh, Sounds True Audio
13. The Eight Human Talents, Gurmukh, HarperCollins
14. The Psychology of Kundalini Yoga, C.G. Jung, Princeton University Press
15. The Secrets to Manifesting Your Destiny, Dr. Wayne Dyer, Nightingale Conant Audio
16. Yoga Basics, Mara Carrico, Owl Books

Cultivate positive healthy relationships and eliminate the negative

We will examine how you can stop other people from aging you. This is how you create an anti-aging lifestyle, and it is based on the belief that you become who you associate with. Your lifestyle concerns how you relate every day to yourself and to others in society. Your job, your friends, your family and the misconceptions everyone has about aging have just as much influence on how fast you age as do your habits. Sadly, growing old and dying before your time is the socially acceptable thing to do.

Theory: Avoid negative social conditioning that may cause premature aging

Negative social conditioning is all around you. When you see the majority of people around you doing things a certain way you start to accept that way as a truth, whether it is or not. Just think that only 100 years ago the concept of air travel was considered impossible. Racial segregation was the law in "the land of the free and the home of the brave." And, the only acceptable place for a woman was in the home. Why did so many intelligent people in the past believe such concepts that are obviously ridiculous today? Deepak Chopra refers to this phenomenon as the Hypnosis of Social Conditioning.

You must become the 100th monkey in the cycle of events that changes the tide of social conditioning on the aging dilemma. Deepak

Chopra in his co-authored audiotape *Living Beyond Miracles* recounts the 100th monkey event. Below is a paraphrase of this story.

"On some island in Asia, researchers introduced sweet potatoes to a group of monkeys. The monkeys loved the potatoes but the dirt that surrounded them made them hard to eat and digest. There was one monkey who accidently dropped her sweet potato into a stream of water and upon retrieving the potato noticed it was much easier to eat and digest. Every day she took her potato to the stream and washed it before eating. There were the monkey critics that thought her potato washing was a waste of time because 'if God wanted potatoes to not be covered with dirt, God would have grown them on trees.' She started feeding her little baby and her husband the washed potatoes. Soon other monkeys started imitating her. It was around the time that the 100th monkey washed its potato that scientists noticed a remarkable phenomenon. These Asian scientists were relaying their observations to other monkey scientists around the world and lo and behold, after that 100th monkey started washing her potato, all the monkeys all over the world started to wash their potatoes as well."

Many of the major social institutions in our society are over-aging you by the hypnosis of social conditioning. Just like the monkey had her critics for being different from the social norm you will have yours. Don't despair, because if you want to keep getting what you're getting, then just keep doing what you're doing. You can look forward to a life that ends decades before it has to, and look and feel old by listening to the critics. Or you can die looking youthful, well into your second century by becoming one of those 100 monkeys that makes a difference in the social consciousness. The choice is yours.

Learn from your parent's ailments; don't repeat them

The majority of ailments and problems you get comes from lifestyle, not from heredity. If your parents had high blood pressure, or as the doctors say, "if high blood pressure runs in your family", then chances are likely you will have it too. The reason may be the lifestyle your family chooses to live. You not only inherit faulty genes from your parents, you also inherit faulty lifestyles. If your family has a history of high blood pressure, then it's more than likely your family probably has a lifestyle that causes high blood pressure. Since you grew up in that family you have possibly developed those same habits of diet, which results in similar medical ailments.

Blaming heredity for many of your lifestyle ailments attempts to place the blame on a gene from your parents and not on yourself. It removes the focus from you to them. Ask a doctor if your parent died of a heart attack does that increase the likelihood that you may have one? The answer is yes. The reason the doctor may give is heart attacks run in your family. As if the little heart attack virus is just running around your family's house waiting for its chance to jump into your body at the appropriate time.

As a lifestyle indicator, your parent's problems are a great clue, but don't accept them as inevitable. Just because your dad died of stomach cancer doesn't mean you will. Use this information to find out what was wrong with his lifestyle. By looking at heredity you are looking at the effect of the problem and not its cause.

The medical forms in doctors offices would serve you better if they asked questions about your parent's lifestyle habits first and then ask about their ailments. This would serve two very important purposes. First, it would provide you with a way to score your parent's lifestyle. Then you could match the lifestyle to the ailments. From this picture you would begin to see a clear picture of cause and effect.

Psychological genetics

Dr. Bernie Segal, M.D., in *Love Medicine & Miracles* states that:

> "Over the years I have found that my patients tend to get the same diseases as their parents and die at the same

age. I think conditioning is at least as much a factor as genetics disposition. I call it psychological genetics, because I've seen people change the scenario once they have been made aware of it. Too many people think they are doomed to reenact their parents' scripts. A nurse told me after one of my lectures, "I think you may have saved my life. I've been waiting to die of cancer, since my mother had it and my father has it. It never occurred to me that I didn't have to have it."

Your friends and family are constant reminders that the majority of the world is aging too fast. If you are not careful, you begin to think, based on what you see, that maybe this is the way it is supposed to be. This is a very dangerous view. If you follow this view, *"that since my father and all my relatives die at or around 65, I will too";* then buy a coffin for your 64th birthday, because you will need it at age 65.

A famous story of psychological genetics is the life and death of Elvis Presley. Elvis loved his mother Gladys dearly. She died on August, 14, 1958 at young at the age of 46 and Elvis was obsessed with the fact that he too might die in his forties. History shows that Elvis Presley died at the age of 42 on August 16, 1977 almost to the day that his mother died. This is the power of psychological genetics.

Constantly improve the way you communicate with your mate

With the small exception of some people at your job, you spend more time with your mate than anyone else. You need the encouragement you get from your mate. You'll ultimately spend the time that keeps you young with your mate, the time to exercise, study, play, and relax. If you do not do some of these activities together, then your lifestyle is in competition with your relationship. Eventually one must go. Nowadays the lawyers call these irreconcilable differences.

Marry the wrong person and they can make your life a living hell. The majority of people marry the wrong person. This fact is easily verified in our divorce statistics. The majority of marriages started today will end in divorce. A stressful marriage followed by a messy divorce ages you. Fortunately, divorcing yourself from the wrong person may in fact add years to your life.

Relationships provide an abundant source of a positive stress that keeps you young. This positive stress is called love. Remember, your state of mind when you first fell in love with your mate? Remember how everything he or she did was cute and funny, and how you could overlook all of their faults? This is the state of energy which when flowing through your body keeps you very youthful. Although love is an emotion, it is something you can create and practice with your mate daily.

It is important to learn how to communication with your mate. Men and women typically have different styles of communication as noted by John Gray PhD, in his book, **Men are from Mars, Women are from Venus**:

> "We mistakenly assume that if our partners love us they will react and behave in certain ways--the ways we react and behave when we love someone. This attitude sets us up to be disappointed again and again and prevents us from taking the necessary time to communicate lovingly about our differences.
>
> Men mistakenly expect women to think, communicate, and react the way men do; women mistakenly expect men to think, communicate, and react the way women do. We have forgotten that men and women are supposed to be different. As a result our relationships are filled with unnecessary friction and conflict."

Therefore, it is important to constantly strive to better understand how to listen and talk to your mate in a style that is effective. The sections that follow provide methods to facilitate this goal.

Learn constructive ways to verbally express your emotions

The need to exercise your love emotion toward your mate is just as important as exercising before each meal to remove toxic waste from your system. You exercise your love emotion toward your mate physically and verbally. Verbally, you exercise your love emotion to create the positive stress necessary to prolong life and slow down the aging process. You exercise by expressing your inner feelings to your mate in a way that relieves you from carrying the frustration and anger toward them that if not expressed verbally may be expressed later in destructive behaviors. Sadly, some couples do not know how to express negative feelings in words. As John Gray says, "men go to their caves and women talk."

A typical scenario might have the woman unloading all of these feelings on her close friend. The male usually keeps these feelings to himself. The couple exists together in form. This is the couple that seemed to have everything right. They have the right house, the right cars, and the right children; and then suddenly they are filing for divorce citing irreconcilable differences. The woman has spent the past 7 years communicating her problems to a friend and the husband has spent the last 7 years in a cave, constipated with negative emotions that are not being expressed in words.

The communication method called "Withholds" provides a means for you to express your feeling to your mate, whether those feelings are positive or negative, in a manner that is loving and consistent. This technique is credited to Dr Alan P. Brauer, M.D and his wife Donna J. Brauer. This couple co-authored the best selling book, *ESO: Extended Sexual Orgasm*. Surprisingly, a major portion of their book is devoted to the art of verbal communication. Listed below is the script you and your mate will follow.

> "To begin the Withholds exercise, say to your partner, in a neutral tone of voice: "(Name), there's something I've withheld from you." Your partner then replies, "Okay. Would you like to tell me?" You say, "Yes." Then share your Withhold. When you are finished, your partner ends the communication cycle by saying "Thank you" and nothing further.

Be sure you use this precise structure. It automatically alerts you to the beginning of the exercise and reminds you both to follow the rules. It announces that a special communication is starting and reminds you to set aside old patterns of reaction that often generate anger and cause arguments. Be sure to announce your Withholds in a neutral, not an emotional, angry, nagging, or sarcastic tone of voice. That way your partner hears the content of your message clearly and won't be distracted by the tone.

Beginning with this opening statement, each partner then spends two or three minutes verbally appreciating the other partner and mentioning any resentments. Or each partner mentions two appreciations and two resentments and then the other mentions two and two. After each appreciation or resentment, the only allowable response is "Thank you." The listening partner agrees to make no other comment until at least thirty minutes after the exercise, and then only with permission. Total time––five minutes a day."

Kiss and make love with your mate often

Physically you exercise your love emotion through physical contact. In her best-selling book, *How to Make Love All the Time*, Dr. Barbara De Angelis prescribes her 30-second kiss. Do this kiss with your mate every day, just as religiously as you brush your teeth. This is not a friendship kiss, you will hold your mate in full embrace for at least 30 seconds before letting go. Zig Ziglar notes that scientists have proved that couples that do this live longer. Dr. De Angelis also notes that couples must make time for regular sex, daily if possible, even if it's a quickie in the morning. The human contact and warmth alone will add years to your life and keep you in a state of physical contentment.

The number one cause of divorce in America is infidelity. If you are constantly communicating verbally and expressing your feelings and emotional needs to your mate--and you are kissing your mate like a lover everyday and having frequent sex, neither mate would have the time, energy or desire to look outside the relationship.

How old would you be if you forgot your age?

How old would you be if you forgot your age? It is the answer to this question that determines your true age, not the calendar. Assume you were a victim of a car accident while traveling across country by yourself. The police could not identify you and your memory was lost. The doctors would have to guess your age. Assuming you followed the principles of this book the doctors might guess your age to be late 20's to early 30's. In reality your chronological age is really 57. As you recuperated, the doctors would have higher expectations on your healing. They would have higher expectations on your progress during physical therapy. Ultimately their higher expectations result in faster recuperation for you based on the Pygmalion principle. The Pygmalion principle states the people perform to expectations. That is why forgetting your age is so important. Expectations for your ability must be based on who you are and not on something as predictable as your next birthday. Richard Bach writes in his book, *Running from Safety*:

> "When you don't believe in birthdays, the idea of aging turns a little foreign to you. You don't fall into trauma over your sixteenth birthday or your thirtieth or the big Five-Oh or the deadly century. You measure your life by what you learn, not by counting how many calendars you've seen. If you're going to have trauma, better it be the shock of discovering the fundamental principle of the universe than some date predictable as next July."

You're too young to be old

In order to live long and stay youthful, you must be responsibly immature. You must resist the urge to act your age. You must live with reckless abandon in a sensible way. Or, as Wayne Dyer states in *You Will See It When You Believe It*, *"You must live your life by the critical inch instead of by the conservative mile."* The conservative mile is to live by a set of rules that makes you polite, civil, and normal. Many of us live by a set of rules that we all instinctively know. If you don't know the rules you can go to any bookstore and buy the runaway best seller *Life's Little Instruction Book Vol I and II*, by H. Jackson Brown Jr., and receive 1028 suggestions, observations and reminders on how to live a happy and rewarding life. They are something like this,

- "be the first to say, hello;
- buy great books even if you don't read them;
- floss your teeth;
- praise in public; criticize in private."

If you master these rules you live a "normal" happy life, with not a whole lot of trouble and you get by. If you only live by the rules and never express your own desires, then this kind of life, in the words of Les Brown the motivational speaker, *"causes us to quietly tip-toe to an early grave."* Some people never truly live life because they are spending so much time learning and living by the rules.

Living by the critical inch usually happens after a tragic life altering event such as a car accident, the death of a loved one, or the false diagnosis of a major illness. This is when the person starts to question the rules and determine what is their purpose on this planet. This is when the person quits the job on Wall Street that was giving them a big paycheck along with marriage problems, alcoholism, and ulcers and goes to an under-developed country to help the village people learn to build houses. This is when the over 50 MBA from Wharton, quits his six-figure job to open that surf shop on the beach. This is living the critical inch versus the conservative mile. Ironically, the people who live by the critical inch, end up with more of the "things" that they thought living life by the "rules" would bring. They end up with more money, happiness, and fulfillment than ever.

It seems like the older we get the more we cling to the rules as our salvation, when it is the rules that ultimately cause you to die twice as fast. It's your wild nature that ultimately causes you to live much longer.

As Dr. Clarissa Pinkola Estes, author of **Women Who Run with the Wolves** states,

> "Wild means natural; being connected to one's instincts; being connected to one's deepest soul. We are domesticated away from that wildness, so we are mild and submissive. We are trained to be 'contained' in a box of life never venturing outside the limits of that box to explore, because that is for the young. So we accept the rule that we must act our age and nothing more."

Instinctively, we all attempt to break out of the box. We know we are young, and yet society is telling us we are old. Society has a label for this syndrome called mid-life crisis. Everything about this label is wrong and negative. A man turns 40 and buys a fancy car, a woman turns 40 and gets out of a dead marriage to live with a younger man, someone quits their job to live their dream, and do we applaud these actions? No we don't applaud these actions––we tell them they're crazy, they are going through a phase, a mid-life crisis. What is happening is our wild nature, to be more than just a person, is trying to escape, and we are told to get back in the box. We are ridiculed, and ostracized for our "childish actions." Most people return to the box. They sell the Corvette and return to the Volvo, they leave the hot steamy young lover, to return to the safe marriage that lacks desire. They give up their dream and return to the rat race of corporate America; all because they are criticized for not acting their age. They quietly tiptoe to that early grave along with everyone else that is "acting their age" and living by the rules. Jump out of the box.

Tina Turner was asked during the filming of a documentary on her life, what made her different from all the other singers of her time and why has she been successful for so many years. Her answer was, *"I kicked and stepped out on the edge, while everyone else stuck to the rules."*

You are entitled to be immature until the day you die. When Bill Gates left Harvard as a freshman to start a computer company catering to the PC (Personal Computer) market, he wasn't being hailed as a genius. At that time, PCs were toys for hobbyists, ranking next to the amateur ham radio. Why leave a sure thing to risk it all on an industry that doesn't even exist? Why leave one of the best schools in America to play with a hobby. Well, 15 years later Mr. Gates is America's wealthiest man. He jumped out of the box.

Your life's ultimate reality is based only on two things: what you think about, and what you do. If you live your life based on a role society has placed on your age, then plan on dying 50 years before you have to and looking extremely old. No, act immature, live your life like there is no tomorrow; because for all you know there may not be a tomorrow. The future is promised to no one; all we have is the present moment. Everything else is just a dream, a hope, a wish, and an illusion of things that might come.

Don't just repeat last years experience

Every day you are a new creature, old things are past away and behold all things are new. II Cor 5:17

Les Brown says that, *"many people die at age 23 and don't get buried until age 65. They are walking dead people."* Without challenge you die a slow death of boredom. Yet life tells you to play it safe. You hear it all the time in our quaint little sayings to each other like, "take it easy; don't work too hard; be careful." Some people are just going through the motions. Just waiting for the game to end. Some workers with 10 years at a particular job don't have 10 years of experience. What they have is one year of experience repeated 10 times.

All things in nature are continually becoming new and you must continually be learning and trying new activities in life; otherwise, you fall victim to becoming obsolete in a world that is continually changing. You must choose to live your life either by living 80 years one year at a time, or by living one year repeated 80 times. Choose the former and you age very slowly. Choose the latter and you age exponentially. The choice is yours.

Do activities that are exciting and exhilarating

One of my favorite stories concerns the late billionaire Malcolm Forbes Jr. who was an avid motorcycle rider. Although he was very active throughout his life and very vital until his death, he still had the appearance of an old man. One day while he and a friend were riding their motorcycles down a long country road they reached an intersection and waited beside a school bus for the light to change. Peering outside the window one of the school kids looked down at Mr. Forbes on the motorcycle and yelled, "hey old man, you're too old to be riding a motorcycle." To which Mr. Forbes replied, "hey young fellah, you're too young not to."

This story illustrates how we allot our time for adventure and excitement to our youth, and resign ourselves to a safe life, as we grow older. It's the very resignation to being safe that helps perpetuate your old age. The thrill of doing something new and exciting stimulates the adrenalin and activates the mind to conquer fear. You must always challenge yourself no matter what your age. You must do something exciting and exhilarating.

Stop telling your age; it is nobody's business

Your age is not the business of any police officer, bouncer, doorman, or election official. All they need to know is if you are of legal age to do the activity. An alternative to placing your age on an identification card is to use universally accepted codes. This provides the business the ability to meet their need to ensure people are of legal age and also protects your confidentially. Codes similar to those below would meet this need.

TD	Teen Driver: Signifies this driver is old enough to have a drivers permit but too young to drive alone.
YD	Young Driver: Signifies that this driver is of legal age to drive but not yet 21.
A	Adult: signifies that this driver is 21 years or older.

Choosing to look decades younger than your actual age may cause you to tell white lies about your age. It is not that your age is something to be ashamed of to the point that you have to lie about it. The sad truth is that society judges you as less valuable as your age increases. In the workplace, society lies to you when it says your age doesn't matter; only your ability. Age discrimination in the work place is running rampant in this era of corporate downsizing.

If you want to be 29 for the rest of your life and can look, act, think, and function as a person that is 29, then you are just as honest in saying you are 29 even if your driver's license says you are 45. The reason you are just as honest is because age comes in two distinct categories: chronological and biological. You are just choosing to state your biological age instead of your chronological age. Your chronological age is the age listed on your driver's license, and your biological age is the shape and upkeep of your physical appearance.

Use your biological age to measure and maximize your life span

The way you choose to measure your age influences how long you may live. A classic example of how this works is the story of the miners trapped in the shaft of a collapsed mine with only a couple of hours of air to breathe. The only miner with a watch counted out the time twice as slow; to give the other men hope that they might have enough air to survive until they got dug out. When the men were finally rescued, all were alive except for the man who counted the time. His death was a true representation of how many of us die. We base our dying time on the measure of birthday time.

Chronological time is how you measure how long you have lived. This time is measured by clocks and calendars in relation to how many times the sun rises in the east and sets in the west. This is an excellent way to measure time for certain purposes such as record keeping. It is a terrible way to measure time if you want to age slower and maximize life span potential because the focus is always on the past.

You must move away from marking your life by calendars and start marking it by the condition of your body. Use your biological age instead of your chronological age. You have no control over the calendar, but you have lots of control over your body. Focusing your energies on what you can control is healthier and more satisfying than trying to beat time that never slows down and moves at the speed of light.

Biological age--The condition of your appearance and health

The Carter Center of Emory University has developed a computer program that provides a health Risk appraisal to calculate your biological age, entitled "Healthier People." This program accepts the lab work numbers from your doctor and asks you questions about your lifestyle to give an estimate of your true biological age. Just imagine visiting your doctor's office and she says, "Based on your test for this year I am pleased to inform you that for the 15th year in a row you have tested and passed the criteria for a 37 year old man. Congratulations!" This is terrific news if your chronological age is really 60 years old. Also, the book **RealAge**, by Michael F. Roizen, M.D., provides a chart to calculate your biological age. If you have Internet access, www.RealAge.com will allow you to take the assessment on-line.

Biological time is a much better way to measure age. It cuts down on all the discrimination and shallowness that comes with measuring people based on when they were born. If a person looks, acts, and feels forty, and has all the biological indicators such as blood cholesterol, correctable eyesight, heart rate, agility, strength, and reflexes of someone forty years of age; then that person deserves the opportunity to perform whatever work a forty year old could perform, even if that person has a chronological age of sixty-five.

For occupations that are physically, emotionally, or mentally demanding and also place the lives of innocent people at risk (e.g. CEO's, police and fire professionals, airline pilots) this type of testing is better and safer than our current system of retiring competent, highly skilled people who can still perform but are retired because they reached a mandatory age. It is a better system because it keeps the experience in the workforce longer. It is a safer system because mandatory testing after age 50 would keep many of these professionals in better physical condition since they know they have to test on a regular basis.

Honor your parents by caring for them in their old age

Deuteronomy, chapter 5 and verse 16, states, *"Honor your parents (remember this is a commandment of the Lord your God); if you do so, you shall have a long, prosperous life."* This is the 5th commandment given to Moses for the people of Israel by God. It is the only commandment from the Ten Commandments that promises a reward if obeyed. That reward is a long life.

The definition of the word "honor" in this text means caring for your parents in old age. There are several social benefits keeping this commandment provides. First, by caring for your parents in their old age you catch a glimpse of problems you may encounter and learn from their ordeal. Secondly, there is the golden rule of what goes around comes around. It is nice to think that when you are old your progeny may honor you.

Bibliography for the 2nd Principle

1. A Fine Romance: The Passage of Courtship from Meeting to Marriage, Judith Sills, Ballantine Press
2. Attracting Terrific People: How to find and keep the people who bring your life joy, Lillian Glass, St. Martin's Press
3. ESO: Extended Sexual Orgasm, Alan & Donna Brauer, Warner Books
4. Keeping the Love You Find, Harville Hendrix, Pocket Books
5. Focus on the Family--call 1-800-AFAMILY
6. How to be Irresistible to the Opposite Sex, Susan Bradley, Loving University Press
7. How to Make Love All the Time, Barbara De Angelis, Dell Publishing
8. How to Stop Worrying & Start Living, Dale Carnegie, Pockets Books
9. Life's Little Instruction Book Vol I and II, H. Jackson Brown Jr., Rutledge Hill Press
10. Live Your Dreams, Les Brown, William Morrow & Co.
11. Living Beyond Miracles, Wayne W. Dyer and Deepak Chopra, Amber-Allen Audio

12. Love Medicine & Miracles, Bernie S. Siegal, Harper Audio
13. Loving Each Other, Leo Buscaglia, Nightingale Conant Audio
14. Making Miracles: Finding Meaning in Life's Chaos, Paul Pearsall, Prentice Hall
15. Men are from Mars, Women are from Venus, John Gray, Harper Collins
16. Reading People: How to Understand People and Predict Their Behavior, Jo-Ellan Dimitrius and Mark Mazzarella, Random House
17. RealAge, Michael F. Roizen, M.D., HarperCollins
18. Running from Safety, Richard Bach, Dell Publishing
19. The Aladdin Factor, Jack Canfield & Mark Victor Hansen, Berkley Press
20. The Beauty Myth, Naomi Wolf, Doubleday
21. The Virtues of Aging, Jimmy Carter, NewStar Publishing
22. Understanding Human Nature, Alfred Adler, One World Oxford
23. What Your Mother Couldn't Tell You & Your Father Didn't Know: Advanced Relationship Skills for Better Communication and Lasting Intimacy, John Gray, Harper Audio
24. Women Who Run with the Wolves, Clarissa Pinkola Estes, Random House
25. You Just Don't Understand: Women and Men in Conversation, Deborah Tannen, Ballantine
26. You'll See it When You Believe It, Dr. Wayne Dyer, William Morrow & Co.

Think and grow healthy, wealthy, and wise

Growing healthy means making the right choices of habit. All of your habits find their origins from your thoughts. William Makepeace Thackeray said, *"we sow a thought and reap an act; we sow an act and reap a habit; we sow a habit and reap a character; we sow a character and reap a destiny."* The risk for mental disorders increases as you approach advanced ages. Research has shown that appropriate habits of thinking can reduce this risk. You will learn these thinking habits to keep your brain healthy.

Growing wise is characterized by making good decisions based on the available information. It is the ability to habitually make good decisions and thus avoid the pitfalls and common accidents of life. Statistically, the fourth leading cause of death is accidents. Therefore, poor habits of thinking can result in you not living out the full number of years. You will learn how to avoid these common accidents.

Growing wealthy is the ability to receive in excess of what you need to survive and invest the surplus for distribution in the future. Being wealthy is the discipline of investing your surplus and then living on the interest. Wealth means more that just money, it is an abundance of anything that is valuable. Thus, you can be wealthy in friendships, wealthy in happiness, and wealthy in influence. You will learn a plan of study to become healthy, wealthy, and wise.

Theory: Your body ages slower when toxic thinking is countered with positive physiology

In his runaway best seller, *Ageless Body Timeless Mind*, Dr. Deepak Chopra documents how toxic chemicals are produced when you use your mind to worry; how the mind produces chemical reactions just by your thoughts. Deepak states,

> "The revolution we call mind body medicine was based on the simple discovery that wherever a thought goes a chemical goes with it. Medicine is just beginning to use the mind body connection for healing, using placebos or dummy drugs to kill pain, to stop excessive gastric secretions in ulcer patients, to lower blood pressure or fight tumors. Since the same inert pill can lead to such totally different responses, we have to conclude the body is capable of producing its own biochemical response once the mind has been given the appropriate suggestion. The pill itself is meaningless, the power that activates the placebo effect is the power of suggestion alone. This suggestion gets converted into the body's intention to cure itself. Therefore why not bypass the deception of the sugar pill and go directly to the intention. If we could effectively trigger the intention not to age, the body would carry it out automatically."

The brain will also write prescriptions based on actions--and actions over-rule the prescription of a thought. So if you have sad thoughts but force yourself to laugh, the brain will produce the drug for joy. If you feel sad, then start to laugh. If you feel scared, then act fearless. Feeling happy causes the brain to produce drugs to make you feel euphoric. Feeling sad causes the brain to produce drugs to make you feel depressed. That is why you can control how you feel by acting the way you want to feel.

The problem is that most people use their brain incorrectly through worry, fear, and guilt, to over-produce chemical reactions that are toxic. Neurologists have learned a great deal about how the mind can produce chemicals. You must use this knowledge to ensure your thinking habits produce the chemicals that keeps your body healthy.

Eliminate erroneous habits of thinking to age slower

"Cancer is not a primary disease; its partly a reaction to a set of circumstances that weaken the bodies defenses."
Dr Bernie S. Siegel, M.D.

"If you're plagued by guilt or worry and find yourself unwittingly falling into the same old self-destructive pattern then you have erroneous zones", says Dr. Wayne Dyer. His book, **Your Erroneous Zones** explains how these erroneous zones cause your emotions to negatively control your life. Let's now focus on how these same erroneous zones (i.e. worry, fear, and procrastination) accelerate the aging process and what you can do to stop it.

Erroneous thinking about the present

Procrastination is using the present moment talking about what you are going to do, but never doing it. Pushing the present into a future that never happens. The exercise plan, the diet, the self-improvement is considered but never attempted. Once procrastination has served its course the person then resorts to either guilt or worry to occupy the rest of his or her time.

Procrastination is the reason most people never live to see age 90. Procrastination is the reason people appear 120 years old by the time they are 70. They never did the things in their life that would have slowed down the aging process. How many people are going to stop smoking, are going to start exercising, are going to go on a diet, are going to go back to school, are going to start that business, or write that book? Procrastination is that road to hell paved with good intentions. It is the thought that "I know what I must do, but I'll do it tomorrow."

To eliminate procrastination you must develop the habit of action. This is the ability to do it now. Plan your work and then work your plan.

Erroneous thinking about the future

When you worry you use your mind to trigger many bio-chemical reactions internally that prematurely ages you from the inside out and may even kill you. Medical evidence proves that worry is a contributing factor for many serious physical ailments such as stroke and heart attacks. Worry is an erroneous habit of thinking.

To eliminate the habit of worry you must develop the habit of planning and goal setting. Worry is fear of the future, and taking the time to plan can reduce this fear.

Jesus points out the folly of worry in Matthew 6:25:

> "So I tell you, don't worry about everyday life--whether you have enough food, drink, and clothes. Doesn't life consist of more than food and clothing? Look at the birds. They don't need to plant or harvest or put food in barns because your heavenly Father feeds them. And you are far more valuable to him than they are. Can all your worries add a single moment to your life? Of course not. And why worry about your clothes? Look at the lilies and how they grow. They don't work or make their clothing, yet Solomon in all his glory was not dressed as beautifully as they are. And if God cares so wonderfully for flowers that are here today and gone tomorrow, won't he more surely care for you? You have so little faith! So don't worry about having enough food or drink or clothing. Why be like the pagans who are so deeply concerned about these things? Your heavenly Father already knows about your needs, and he will give you all you need from day to day if you live for him and make the Kingdom of God your primary concern. So don't worry about tomorrow, for tomorrow will bring its own worries. Today's trouble is enough for today."

Erroneous thinking about the past

Guilt is erroneous thinking about things that have happened in the past. It's making you feel bad for what you could have done. People use guilt to make you tip a little more, or buy something you really didn't want to.

To eliminate guilt thinking you must develop a forgettory[3]. A forgettory is the ability to learn from and then forget the past. There is nothing you can do to change what has already happened to you. Learn from your past and then move on by using that information to better plan for the future.

Avoid the common accidents of life that age you prematurly

Morris Landis, a very successful investor, explains the need to avoid the common accidents of life with a story called the Potholes of Life.

> "Think of life as a journey and your destination is success. Along the way you must take care to not fall into the potholes of life. The bigger the pothole the more damage it can cause to your car and the harder it is to get out of the hole. Many people think that falling into the potholes is a necessary part of the journey. That is not true. All falling into a pothole will do is delay arriving at your destination and waste good money on repairs that could have been used for other purposes. The real loss from falling into a pothole is time. The time it takes for you to get out of a hole can never be returned no matter how good your intentions. In fact, if there are several persons attempting to get to the same destination, while you are trying to get out of that hole, your competition will be miles ahead of you by the time you get out. The best way to avoid falling into potholes is to know where they are and go around them. Many potholes are very obvious to a person that has traveled on that same road

---

[3] Word coined by Dr. Wayne Dyer, "Your Sacred Self", HarperCollins Publishers, 1995

before you. Think of that person as a road map, one who can point out the detours along the way and the roads to avoid, so that you don't have to make the mistakes that eat up valuable time on your journey."

These potholes not only take your time and money; they are also a key source of stress and aging. Aging from potholes can make you become bitter and cynical towards life since the accident occurred while you were traveling toward success. The attitude develops that this wouldn't have happened if I were just content with my lot in life. The worn look of experience on a person's face might lead to thoughts of character and maturity but the truth is this aging need not have occurred.

Listed below are 17 common mistakes to avoid in your lifetime.
1. Learning by mistakes versus learning from other people's experience
2. Neglecting to wear seat belts when in a moving vehicle
3. Marriage before emotional maturity is reached
4. Poor selection of a marriage partner
5. Lack of written goals
6. Failure to start saving for retirement at an early age
7. Failure to improve interpersonal relationship skills
8. Failure to have a written will
9. Failure to choose to be happy
10. Lack of adequate home owner's or renter's insurance
11. Lack of adequate liability and health insurance
12. Choosing a career based on money instead of what you love
13. Starting addictive habits of sex, drugs, alcohol and cigarettes at an early age
14. Purchasing a home before you can save the down payment
15. Living on credit to support status symbols
16. Choosing career success over family success
17. Trusting the opinion of others over your own

Determine the cause of the effect

In this cause and effect world, we have mistakenly labeled the effect as the cause of aging and death. For example, when a smoker dies of lung cancer we label the cause of death cancer. The real cause of death was smoking and the effect was lung cancer. By labeling the cause as the effect, it allows you to kid yourself in the belief that the death was somehow just part of the process of life, out of your control. The following table further illustrates this point.

Top 10 Killers According to Effect of Disease		Top Nine Killers According to Actual Cause Due to Lifestyle[4]	
Heart Disease	720,000	Tobacco	400,000
Cancer	505,000	Diet and Activity	300,000
Strokes	144,000	Alcohol	100,000
Accidents	92,000	Microbial Agents	90,000
Pulmonary Disease	87,000	Toxic Agents	60,000
Pneumonia, Influenza	80,000	Firearms	35,000
Diabetes	48,000	Sexual Behavior	30,000
Suicide	31,000	Motor Vehicles	25,000
Liver Disease	26,000	Illicit Drug Use	20,000
AIDS	25,000		

The next time you hear of someone dying, notice what the people say. Nine times out of 10 they state the effects, not the cause. It is time for you to take responsibility for your own long life. Many people age before their time from bad habits. Learn the rules that allow you to live a very long time while aging slower and feeling extremely healthy. Proper thinking habits allow you to make lifestyle decisions that avoid or substantially reduce the risk of an early demise due to a poor lifestyle.

Learning from others is the best way

Life gives lessons--and until you pass those lessons you have to continue retaking the tests. In many ways these tests are open book exams; but

---

[4] Journal of the American Medical Association, McGinnis, J.M. et al. Actual causes of death in the United States. Issue 270:2207-2212, 1993.

few people ever bother to open the book. They want to learn it on their own.

Who would you want performing open-heart surgery on your little baby? Someone who has studied the philosophy of open-heart surgery, and received straight A's from John Hopkins Medical School, attended all the current lectures on open heart surgery and is considered one of the brightest open-heart surgery prospects, but has yet to perform a single surgery on a living human. Or would you want someone who scored C's at a small-unknown medical school, but has performed over 100 completely successful open-heart surgeries on patients your child's age? The answer is obvious; experience always wins over potential, no matter how outstanding that potential is.

You want experience that produces results. There are so many books and tapes and seminars in the market by people who are and are not producing good results. Your key is to focus only on the authors that produce results. Some books sound good but the results are questionable. You need more than a good sound; you need results. These results must be evident in either the author's life or by the people following his or her advice. If neither is present then don't waste your time with their nice sounding ideas.

Trial and error is a necessary way to invent new things but a lousy way to live life. Many things you will attempt in life have already been done by millions of people. The better ways to do things are public record. That's how professions such as psychiatry, sociology, and dentistry were established. The best of the findings were recorded and improved upon over time. Failure when trying to discover something new is good in the laboratory only. The often heard quote from Thomas Edison when asked how it felt to fail 10,000 times before inventing the light bulb was, *"I did not fail 10,000 times I just found 10,000 ways not to make a light bulb."* You don't want to find 10,000 ways to not make your marriage work, or raise your family, or succeed in your career. You want to do it right the first time.

The McDonald's corporation franchises illustrate the value of learning from successful models. If you buy a McDonald's you are required to do business in the McDonald's way, no deviation. There are literally thousands of McDonald's throughout the world and all of them are successful--every single one. If you purchase a McDonald's and follow the rules outlined in your franchise documentation, you most likely will succeed. This is the beauty of learning from other people's experience instead of finding out the hard way.

Reduce your risk of Alzheimer's by doing brain exercises

Your brain needs exercise in order to function properly. Unlike your other organs that are stimulated by purely physical activity and nutrition, your brain is nourished by learning and exercised by thinking. The more you think the better and longer your brain functions. Medical studies are proving that poor thinking skills powerfully predict the onset of Alzheimer's disease.

"Alzheimer's is a thinking disease," said David Snowdon, associate professor of preventive medicine at the University of Kentucky in Lexington. "it seems plausible that if you can develop your thinking ability, your thinking reserve, you might be protected against thinking diseases later on."

"The way you use words reflects a fundamental way you do your thinking," he said. "Language may be a marker of general mental ability." Snowdon's study appears in today's edition of the Journal of American Medical Association. For reasons that will soon become clear, he calls it the "nun study." Alzheimer's is an incurable, degenerative brain disease. It tends to afflict older people and is characterized by the loss of memory, language ability, and mental skills.

Researchers are studying the 678 nuns of the School of Sisters of Notre Dame in Milwaukee, who have all agreed to donate their brains to a federally funded research study on the effects of Alzheimer's disease on the brain. As a start, the academics compared 93 nuns' ability to write essays when they were in their

20's--an average of 58 years ago--and whether they had developed Alzheimer's. They found that weak language skills in early life were closely linked to the development of disease later on.

When the scientists conducted autopsies on the brains of 25 nuns who had died--10 of whom had Alzheimer's-- the correlation between abundant neurofibrillary tangles, which are the lesions of Alzheimer's disease, and early language weaknesses was equally powerful.

"Ninety percent of those with Alzheimers had low language ability vs. 13 percent without Alzheimer's who had low linguistic ability," Snowdon said.

There are four exercises that keep your brain healthy and vital for your 120-year life span. The first exercise is to listen and watch educational tapes. The second exercise is to read books. The third exercise is to write journal or diary entries of your thoughts. The fourth exercise is to learn to read and play music or to speak and read in a second language.

Listen and watch educational tapes

Audiocassettes are an excellent way to obtain knowledge while you are doing other things. Transform your car and the public transportation system into temples of learning. Today, most books can be purchased on audiocassette tape. Listen to these tapes during your commute to and from work each day. With this method you can listen to 3 books a week.

Writing in a journal or diary

Writing a diary or journal of your thoughts forces your brain to translate your mental thoughts into written words and sentences. Carry a journal in your pocket or bag wherever you go. Whenever you get an idea or thought or even information you need, but don't need to remember, write it down. George Bernard Shaw once wrote, "*I have become rich and famous by thinking just a couple times a week."* You may not become rich and famous, but the habit of writing your thoughts gives your brain the exercise it needs to take you into a 120-year life span. It also helps you to become a better thinker because the way you write is a reflection of the way you think. A clear writing style reflects clear thinking.

Read and play music or read and write a foreign language

Reading music is a neuro-locomotive exercise that requires the ability to translate a musical symbol into a physical action. The ability to read music affects both sides of the brain. The left side of the brain is intrigued by the technical translations of symbols into movement. The right side of the brain is stimulated by the creative rhythms that the resulting sounds make. Find an instrument you like to play and learn to read the sheet music at once. Practice this instrument daily and you may begin to see your creative powers of mind over matter greatly enhanced as your musical skills increase. These same benefits are obtained by learning to speak and write in a second language.

Read books

Reading books forces the brain to translate symbols into words and then words into ideas for you to think about. The book *How to Read A Book*, by Mortimer J. Adler teaches you how get the most out of every book you read.

Begin to carry a book in your pocket or bag wherever you go. We now live in a time of lines. You have to wait for everything from getting food for lunch to a dental appointment. While you are waiting, just pull out that book and start reading. This method allows you to read about 2 books a month while waiting in lines.

In addition to your reading while waiting in lines, set aside a regular time to read. A good habit is to set aside 30 minutes a day for reading. This allows you to read 1 book a week, or 52 books a year, or 520 books a decade. If these books are about making money, or staying healthy, or having a better relationship, do you think they will have an effect on your life? Do you think the person that reads 520 books about how to make money is going to have a significant advantage over the person that never reads such books? The answer is obvious. Make the time and exercise your brain by reading daily.

A plan of study to become healthy, wealthy and wise

Brian Tracy notes that the average person that graduates from high school reads only one book per year and that book is usually fiction. It is with books that you begin to slow the aging process in your brain by filling it with the information necessary to achieve this goal. You cannot read just any book. You must read the books that improve your thinking ability and increase your faith in yourself and your ability to age slower and live healthier. Reading must become your life-long habit. You can absorb the knowledge that may have taken the author 10 years to acquire in a matter of days. You begin to receive the benefits of knowledge that might have taken you 10 years or more to figure out on your own.

Clearly, with so much information on the market and so many areas to explore, the task of knowing where to begin could be overwhelming. Therefore, focus on the following 4 areas: your love life, your health, your personal finances, and your career. In the sections that follow you are introduced to books that are proven to produce good results. This is a good place for you to begin in your educational quest.

1. Make A study of love

Everything you ever want or do depends on other people--getting a job, marrying, raising your children, buying a house--everything depends on others. The more skill you have in your ability to understand the rules of getting along with others the better quality of life you have.

Here are 7 books to read that improve your ability to love
1. *Are You The One For Me?, by Dr. Barbara De Angelis*
2. *First Corinthians Chapter 13, by Saint Paul the Apostle*
3. How To Win Friends and Influence People, by Dale Carnagie
4. *Loving Each Other, by Leo Busciallia*
5. *Man's Search for Meaning, by Victor Frankel*

6. *You Can Heal Yourself, by Louise L. Hay*
7. *Your Erroneous Zones, by Dr. Wayne Dyer*

2. Make A study of your health

After the ability to love and be loved, there is nothing of greater value than your health. Become a student of physical education. Your books must range from nutrition to medicine; from vitamins to exercise. Here are 7 books to read that improve your health.

1. *Dr. Mollen's Anti-Aging Diet, by Dr. Art Mollen*
2. *Eat to Win, by Dr Robert Haas*
3. *Eight Weeks to Optimum Health, by Dr. Andrew Weil*
4. *Fit for Life, by Harvey and Marilyn Diamond*
5. *Sugar Busters, by Dr. H. Leighton Steward*
6. *The Education of a Body Builder, by Arnold Schwarzenegger*
7. *The Road Less Traveled, by Dr. M. Scott Peck*

3. Make a study of your vocation

After your relationships and your health are in order your next priority is your vocation. We live in demanding times. The law of the jungle is in effect––only the strong survive. If you want to stay employed in the 21st century, you had better be very knowledgeable and skilled at what you do. Become so confident of your skills that you are doing your employer a favor by staying there instead of starting your own business. If your skills are not at that level then watch out. No matter how skilled you are, you could still be unemployed because you are too old and making too much money. That is why it is important to keep your skills at the leading edge of your industry. You must read at least 1 book a week (on company time and expense) at your job about your field and subscribe to at least 1 trade magazine (at company expense) in your field. If possible, have your employer send you to school and training (on company time) to get industry recognized certifications. By doing these things you become too valuable to downsize. Even if you are downsized, you have the skills to quickly get another job or make it on your own.

Here are 6 books to read to improve your vocation.

1. *How to be a Successful Executive, by J. Paul Getty*
2. *Lead the Field, By Earl Nightingale*
3. *The Art of Exceptional Living, by Jim Rohn*
4. *Trump: The Art of the Deal, by Donald Trump*
5. *Unlimited Power, by Anthony Robbins*
6. *What Color is Your Parachute, Richard N. Bolles*

4. Make a study of money and finance

You must master the ability to make more money and keep more of the money you make. We live in a world that discriminates because of age. As you live well into your 90's and beyond it is rare to find a person that is employed by someone else. The only person that comes to mind is George Burns, and in many ways he was employed as a novelty of old age. There are few people like George Burns who are in demand for employment after the age of 90.

Therefore, you must learn how to save money, because it is this money that sustains you probably for the 50 years of your retirement (assuming you retire at age 70). If done right, you will be able to live very comfortably and affluently without ever having to work for money again. Many of us have no problem making money. Our problem is we spend more than we make. As a nation we are paying taxes just to pay the interest on the national debt. The ability to master your finances is a skill and art that must be acquired. Here are 7 books to read to improve your financial knowledge.

1. *How to Get Rich and Stay Rich, by Fred Young*
2. *Rich Dad, Poor Dad, Robert T. Kiyosaki*
3. *The 401(k) Millionaire, by Knute Iwaszko*
4. *The Millionaire Next Door, Thomas J. Stanley*
5. *The Richest Man in Babylon, by George S. Clason*
6. *Think and Grow Rich, by Napolean Hill*
7. *Wealth Without Risk, by Richard Givens*

Focus your thoughts on living longer, aging slower, and feeling better

"You become what you think about", is an important rule to obey in order to age slower. You must begin to form the habit of thinking about aging slower and living healthier. The more you think about anything the more your brain finds ways to make the thought a reality. Jesus said, *"All things are possible to those who believe."* This even means the ability to live much longer and age much slower. The reason many people up to this point age too fast and die too young is because that is what they see everyone else doing.

Bibliography for the 3rd principle

1. Ageless Body, Timeless Mind, Deepak Chopra, Random House Inc.
2. Goals, Zig Ziglar, Simon & Schuster
3. How to Read a Book, Mortimer J. Adler, Simon & Schuster
4. I've Forgotten Everything I learned In School, Marilyn Vos Savant, St. Martin's Press
5. Lead the Field, Earl Nightingale, Nightingale Conant
6. Man's Search for Meaning, Victor Frankel, Simon & Schuster
7. Possibility Thinking: What great thing would you attempt, if you knew you could not fail?, Dr. Robert H. Schuller, HarperCollins
8. Six Thinking Hats, Edward de Bono, Brown Little & Co.
9. Super Self: Doubling your personal effectiveness, Charles J. Givens, DIANE Publishing
10. The 7 Habits of Highly Effective People, Stephen R. Covey
11. The Greatest Secret in the World, Og Mandino, Bantam Doubleday Dell Publishing
12. The Magic of Thinking Big, David Schwartz, Simon & Schuster
13. The Power of Positive Thinking, Norman V. Peale, Random House Inc.
14. The Psychology of Achievement, Brian Tracy, Simon & Schuster Audio
15. The Psychology of Winning: 10 qualities of a total winner, Denis E. Waitley, Berkley Publishing
16. Think and Grow Rich, Napoleon Hill, Fawcett Press

17. Think Big, Ben Carson, Zondervan Publishing
18. Unlimited Power, Anthony Robbins, Simon & Schuster
19. We Live Too Short and Die Too Long: How to Achieve and Enjoy Your Natural 100-Year-Plus Life Span, Walter M. Bortz II, Bantam
20. What Color is Your Parachute, Richard Nelson Bolles, Ten Speed Press
21. Your Erroneous Zones, Wayne W. Dyer, Harper Publishers
22. Your Sacred Self, Dr. Wayne Dyer, HarperColling Publishers

Invest more on yourself than you do on your job and posessions

As you approach advanced years, you may not be able to find work because of age discrimination; or you may no longer desire to work your entire life. Therefore it is incumbent on you to have enough money invested to meet all your needs, wants, and desires for the 50 years of your retirement (assuming you retire at the age of 70). This principle examines ways to spend the money you earn to maximize the odds of having a massive store of wealth well before you are ready to retire. It will also examine ways to ensure that your mental, physical and emotional health is as strong and vital at 120 years as it is during your prime years.

You will learn a method of living on less than you earn and investing the difference on yourself and others. Clearly if you are already having problems living on all that you earn right now, the prospect of living on less sounds unrealistic. Ironically, the reason you are probably having problems making ends meet with your current income has little to do with the amount of money coming in, the problem is the allocation of the money towards expenses.

You are asked to live on 70 percent of the income you produce and invest the other 30 percent in the following distribution. Ten percent is placed in a long-term investment that you never touch until the interest can support all your expenses. Ten percent is spent on yourself and family in the area of self-improvement, buying educational books, tapes, training, seminars, classes, health club memberships, and personal grooming. Ten percent of your gross pay is given to the church or charity. The remaining 70 percent is spent on your bills. Regardless of your circumstances, strive towards living on 70 percent of your paycheck and watch that paycheck grow.

Living beyond your means accelerates aging in several ways. First the money spent on things you can't afford takes away time and money that could have been used to improve your mind, body, and spirit. Also, aging is accelerated from the worrying associated with how to pay the bills.

Morris Landis uses the Pothole story to illustrate the importance of investing more on you than on your possessions--specifically, when young people attempt to purchase a house they cannot afford before investing in themselves first.

"Owning a house you really can't afford is a pothole. As a young person your greatest asset is your mind and your ability to work hard. If you invest your money in your mind, find your vocation and work really hard, you greatly increase the odds that you will be successful and will have money working for you and not the other way around. If you buy a house right now while you still don't know what you want out of life you may spend a great deal of your time fixing the house when it breaks, paying off the mortgage, trying to sell it if you need to move, possibly losing a great deal of money, if the market changes. Most of all you are losing the freedom and time you could use to fill your mind with knowledge, teaching you how to do your job better and become a better person. Most of that money goes into your house. In many ways that house is a very big asset you must drag around with you in all the decisions you want to make concerning what you want to do with your time and life."

Theory: Where you spend your money reflects what you most desire; therefore, desire to constantly improve your mind, spirit and body.

Throughout this book you have been encouraged to purchase books, tapes, the best health care, health club memberships, and a host of other items. This is what investing more on you than on your job or possessions means. The truest measure of what you value is easily determined by where you spend your money. As Jesus said, *"Where your money is, so is your heart also."*

If you truly value health, wealth, wisdom, and love, then a large portion of your income must be spent on healthy foods, health club memberships, educational tapes and books, long-term investments, and donations to charity. The irony in this kind of spending plan is you eventually have more money to spend than you ever need. You can afford to buy the best things in life versus struggling to afford the nice things in life at the expense of your own physical, mental, and social development.

Make money your servant, not your master

The reason you must place 10 percent of your pay in an investment you will not spend until it can support all your living expenses, is to have a store of wealth to support all your needs when you are older. Pay yourself first is the rule to becoming wealthy. The money that you don't spend and invest is similar to a pecan tree farmer that keeps a portion of his crop for planting the next season. If the farmer planted just one seed, that tree may take 10 years or more before it grows big enough to bear abundant fruit. During that time it must be properly cared for so that it can grow big and produce the maximum amount of fruit. When it does bear fruit, that one seed now produces hundreds and maybe thousands of pecans each year. Disciplined saving is analogous to planting a forest instead of planting a single tree. In the span of 15 to 30 years this forest will produce enough pecans to allow you to retire on the fruit from your trees. This is how compound interest works.

Albert Einstein called compound interest the eighth wonder of the world. The power of compound interest allows money to work for you night and day, producing more money that works for you night and day.

Over a period of 15 to 30 years you can become financially independent and live on the interest from your investments. The earlier you start this habit the better. The table below illustrates the consequences of delaying this investment strategy. This example comes from Knute Iwaszko and Brian O'Connell's bestseller, *The 401K Millionaire*. In this example we have two investors Bob and Beth. Both are 65-year-old computer account executives. Bob waited until age 35 to invest in his 401(k). He invested $3000 per year annually for the first 10 years and then never invested another penny. Beth waited until she was 46 to begin investing and to try catching up with Bob, invested $3000 every year until her retirement. Beth contributed twice as much of her own money than Bob--$60,000 versus $30,000--and still fell short of Bob's retirement earnings by about $175,000. That's why it is important to start early.

Age	Bob's Cumulative Investment	Total Value at 10 Percent Annual Return	Beth's Cumulative Investment	Total Value at 10 Percent Annual Return
36	$3,000	$3,168		
37	6,000	$6,667		
38	9,000	10,533		
39	12,000	14,407		
40	15,000	19,521		
41	18,000	24,732		
42	21,000	30,490		
43	24,000	36,850		
44	27,000	43,876		
45	30,000	51,638		
46		57,045	$3,000	$3,168
47		63,018	6,000	$6,667
48		69,617	9,000	10,533
49		76,907	12,000	14,407
50		84,960	15,000	19,521
51		93,856	18,000	24,732
52		103,685	21,000	30,490
53		114,542	24,000	36,850
54		126,536	27,000	43,876
55		139,786	30,000	51,638

56		154,424	33,000	60,212
57		170,594	36,000	69,685
58		188,457	39,000	80,149
59		208,191	42,000	91,710
60		229,992	45,000	104,481
61		254,075	48,000	118,589
62		280,680	51,000	134,174
63		310,070	54,000	151,392
64		342,539	57,000	170,412
65		378,407	60,000	191,424
Total	$30,000	$378,407	$60,000	$191,424

Many people pay everyone else first and then pay themselves last if there is anything left. These are the 97 percent of the population that at age 65 are in need of public assistance. Investing 10 percent of your earnings over a 10-year period equals one year's salary. Practiced over a working lifetime you can easily save 5 times your current salary. A person making $25,000 a year at age 20 can save over a $1,000,000 at the time of retirement. Again quoting Knute Iwaszko and Brian O'Connell from *The 401K Millionaire*,

> "Many younger investors complain that they don't make enough money to participate in a 401(k) plan. I wonder what they'd say if they knew how easy it was to earn over $1 million for retirement by putting away a little over $100 per month.
>
> Take the case of Buddy, a 25-year-old truck driver who makes about $25,000 per year. Buddy says he's got a new convertible to pay off and about $500 in rent a month. But if Buddy stashed away only 6 percent of his salary--about $125 per month--and got a 50 percent company match and a modest 8 percent return from his investments, he would earn $1.1 million by the time he turns 65. And if Buddy stocked away 8 percent of his salary (or $167 per month), he'd reap 1.4 million

by the time he reached 65. A 10 percent or 12 percent investment return on either sum would earn Buddy about $2 million by retirement. All of this on a $25,000 salary."

Investing early, often, and not spending the principle or interest until it can support your lifestyle is how you make money your servant. Sadly, most people live their entire life working for money. They spend all they make and never take advantage of the power of compound interest. If you have to go to work in the morning because you need the money then money is your master. Disobey your master and you can find yourself out on the street, hungry and cold. If your investments support your lifestyle and you work because you choose to, then you are the master of money.

Make it your goal to make money serve you. If you are reading this book and under the age of 21, then make it your goal to master money by the age of 40 much like Benjamin Franklin did. Following the plan of living on 70% of your income you can reach this goal of financial independence in 20years if you work really hard. Even if you are 70 or 80 by the time you reach this goal, you still have another 40 to 50 years of life ahead of you. Don't leave this planet until you reach this goal. Jesus said in Matthew 6:24, *"No person can serve two masters. For you will hate one and love the other, or be devoted to one and despise the other. You cannot serve both God and money."*

Divest yourself from the need to have things own you

All unhappiness is caused by attachment. The Buddha

This is not a discourse on the virtues of poverty or austerity. Material affluence is very important in your quest to live a long and happy life. In fact it is necessary. The vitality of youth is usually lost right after high school as people choose to believe that a good life is a life filled with the most stuff. It's all this stuff that weighs you down. Buddha said that if you want to really have the good things in life you must be willing to detach yourself from wanting to have them. It is the secret to having all the stuff you want without having all the negative consequences that are associated with owning them.

Stay out of consumer debt

The proper way to have lots of stuff without the negative stress is through owning. Owning things eliminates negative stress, and in fact produces positive stress. Remember when your old car got into that fender bender and you didn't care if you ever fixed it because you owned it? Owning happens when you pay cash. It's the security in knowing what you have is yours because it's paid for.

Many people say eat, drink, and be merry on credit cards because tomorrow we may die. What happens if you don't die? What happens if you're still around? Worry happens! Worry over how am I going to pay for the "eat, drink, and be merry" attitude of yesterday. Some people only get the picture after it's too late. They are old before their time at 70 and there are more bills than life in front of them. Of 100 people in the United States that are 20 years old today, only 3 percent will be able to retire comfortably by the age of 65. This 3 percent are the few who knew. They knew that eat, drink, and be merry for tomorrow we die; was really pay cash today, for tomorrow we live.

If you are already in debt then you must immediately begin a plan to get out of debt. Think of each loan, as a chain of slavery and your goal is to become free. Solomon, former king of Israel writes in Proverbs 22:7, *"that the rich rule over the poor and the borrower is the servant to the lender."* Take an accounting of all your outstanding loans. Note the balance due, the monthly payment amount, and the number of payments remaining. Then take the loan with the smallest balance and pay that loan off as quickly as possible. Whenever you get a windfall of money place some of it towards that loan. Once that loan is paid off then proceed to accelerate the payoff of the loan with the next smallest balance. Continue this process until all loans are paid off in full.

If you are in debt because you have the habit of spending more than you earn using credit cards, then avoid debt consolidation loans. These loans allow you to consolidate all your high-interest loans into one lower-interest loan that is paid off over a longer period of time. This lowers your monthly payments and provides a larger cash flow. The problem occurs when the debt consolidation loan pays off your credit cards and you use those cards again and go even deeper into debt. Debt consolidation loans only work if you have developed the discipline and maturity to live within your means.

Invest in your continuing education every year

As you grow older make sure you continuously invest in your education to remain employable. Many people consider education a one-time process reserved for the young. Fifteen years out of high school or college and their skills and knowledge become obsolete and they become filled with anxiety over job cuts every time the economy has a downturn. The fear of being replaced by a younger, lower paid and better-educated person always looms over their head. This is unnecessary mental stress that prematurely ages them. It is also unnecessary stress, since by choosing to keep their education up-to-date they can have the advantage of experience and education to justify their higher income and make them too valuable to downsize.

The reason you must give 10 percent of your pay for self-improvement is to allow you to grow into higher income brackets. This is the seed principle of ever increasing your store of knowledge to make you more valuable to the marketplace. It forces you to focus on the fact that you must return a portion of your paycheck back to the person that provided the paycheck in the first place. This is why some people continue to grow their income every year, while others don't. You are becoming more valuable because of constant self-development. If you cannot afford the better things in life, it is not because they are too expensive, it's because you can't afford them. Investing in yourself makes you become more valuable in the marketplace and allows you to demand and eventually receive a higher income.

Give to charity and invoke the aid of spiritual law

The reason you must give 10 percent of your pay to charity is to gain the aid of spiritual forces and to improve the lives of those less fortunate than you. The bible challenges you to see if you can give at least 10 percent of your gross pay to God first, and then trust in God to meet your needs on the remaining 90 percent. This challenges you to prove your faith by putting your money where your faith is. In Malachi 3:10, God supplies the challenge,

> "Bring all the tithes (10 percent of your pay) into the storehouse, that there will be enough food in my Temple. If you do says the Lord Almighty, I will will open the windows of heaven for you. I will pour out a blessing so great you won't have enough room to take it in! Try it! Let me prove it to you! Your crops will be abundant, for I will guard them from insects and disease. Your grapes will not shrivel before they are ripe, says the Lord Almighty. Then all nations will call you blessed, for your land will be such a delight, says the Lord Almighty."

This is a direct challenge from God. Take the test, and see if you can beat God. If you are not religious then give 10 percent to charity. This principle works but it takes faith to believe it will happen. And the point of the challenge is to prove your faith. This form of sacrifice allows your mind to focus on the fact that you must help others and your getting becomes less selfish.

Bibliography for the 4th Principle

1. Beating the Street, Peter Lynch, Simon & Schuster
2. Buffettology, Mary Buffett, Rawson Associates
3. Dollars & Sense: What the Bible Says about you and Your Money, Larry Burkett, Barbour Publishing
4. Get Rich & Stay Rich, Fred Young, Fell Publishers
5. How to be a Successful Executive, J. Paul Getty, Playboy Publishing
6. How to be Rich, J. Paul Getty, Playboy Publishing
7. How to Get Rich and Stay Rich, Fred J. Young, with Beryl W. Sprinkel, Frederick Publishers, Incorporated

8. Prosperity Consciousness: How to tap your unlimited wealth, Fredric Lehrman, Simon & Schuster Audio

9. Rich Dad, Poor Dad, Robert T. Kiyosaki, Sharon L. Lechter, Warner Books,

10. Seven Strategies for Wealth and Happiness, Jim Rohn, Prima Publishing

11. Swim with the Sharks, Harvey Mackay, Foreword by Kenneth Blanchard, Random House, Incorporated

12. The 401K Millionaire, Knute Iwaszko and Brian O'Connell, Villard Books

13. The Art of Exceptional Living, Jim Rohn, Simon & Schuster Audio

14. The Instant Millionaire: A Tale of Wisdom & Wealth, Mark Fisher, New World Library

15. The Intelligent Investor, Benjamin Graham, HarperCollins Publishing

16. The Millionaire Next Door, Thomas J. Stanley, William D. Danko, Pocket Books

17. The Richest Man in Babylon, George S. Clason, Hawthorn/ Dutton New York

18. The Warren Buffett Way: Investment strategies of the world's greatest investor, Robert G. Hagstrom, Jr., John Wiley & Sons, Incorporated

19. The Wealthy Barber, David Chilton, Prima Press

20. Trump: The Art of the Deal, Donald Trump, Random House

21. Wealth in a Decade, Brett Machtig, Irwin Publishing

22. Wealth Without Risk, Charles J. Givens, Simon & Schuster

PRINCIPLE #5

Exercise before eating and thoroughly flush your system

M any people are dying much too early because they are not getting rid of toxic waste in their body fast enough. In a perfect world, your body would use everything you eat and nothing toxic would ever enter your system. If your body didn't need the nutrients, it would store them for later use. In essence, your body would be a total energy machine, converting everything into energy. This is not how your body works. It extracts the good from the food and discards the bad, which is what you must do in every area of your life. The more efficiently you convert the food to liquid and expel the waste, the less work your body does, the longer you live, and the slower you age.

Theory: People age prematurly because they are not getting rid of toxic waste in their body fast enough.

The white blood cells in your immune system protect your body from all infections and germs. Once the food you have digested becomes waste, it resides in the lower intestines and bladder until it is released. While it is in the body in sufficient amounts, the immune system must stand guard to ensure that none of that waste seeps through the linings of the bladder or intestines. Once the waste is expelled, the immune system can work on other things. The waste weakens the effectiveness of your immune system since it takes it away from doing other things. As you age, the walls of the bladder and intestines start to deteriorate (polyps and bladder infections) causing the immune system to work harder. Just like all the other systems in your body, the immune system's resources are limited. You can only breathe so much air in one breath, the heart can only pump so much blood, and so forth. As your immune system is called to stand guard over the waste, it does not have full strength to work on other infections that attack your body.

To illustrate this point, imagine a truck storing toxic waste traveling down the turnpike and crossing state lines to dump this waste. As the truck approaches each state, the state police for that state assign two cars to follow the truck until it exits the state. If that truck were to ever crash and spill the waste, hundreds of people would be needed in the clean-up effort and the turnpike would be closed. The police that are following this waste truck cannot do other work like giving speeding tickets or stopping drug traffic. They must observe and guard this truck. This is what takes place inside your body. Immune system cells that could rest or do other work must guard this waste. Suppose there is a traffic jam and the truck can only travel 20 miles an hour instead of the normal 65 miles per hour. This means the assigned state police cars must spend more time guarding this truck and the likelihood of it having a problem in that state has increased because it is spending more time getting to the destination.

Now that you understand how the toxic waste theory works, here is how to use it to live longer. Eliminate the waste from your system as quickly as possible. This is done by doing four things: maintaining a proper diet, drinking plenty of water, eating a healthy diet which contains plenty of fiber, and exercising before each meal. It was Jay Leno of the Tonight Show who said, *"a high-fiber diet may increase your life span 20 years, but 15 of those years will be spent on the toilet."* There is an element of truth in this joke.

Drink enough purfied water to flush your system

Urination is a process to eliminate waste from your system. It is an excellent indicator of the level of toxic waste in your body. If you are drinking enough water daily and taking vitamins, you will urinate in three different colors during the course of the day: yellow, green and clear. Your goal is to urinate clear at least once a day. This nutrition plan requires you to drink a minimum of 2 quarts of water per day and recommends you drink 4 quarts of water per day. The last section of this chapter provides a 7-day program that guides you on when to drink and how much to drink to achieve this goal.

Clear Urine Color

Clear urine means that your body is fully saturated with water and your urinary tract and bladder are free of toxic waste. Your body processed the contents of your digestive system up to this point and produced no toxic waste. Those armed guard cells of the immune system can take a rest and regroup their strength. You have achieved a goal that few people rarely attain. This is a significant event of the day. If you drink enough water during the day you may be able to repeat it again before you go to sleep. You will still be eating food throughout the day and creating more toxic waste. Therefore, your next urine after clear might tend towards yellow.

Yellow Urine Color

Yellow is the only color that many people ever see in their urine. They never drink enough water in a day to make it clear. Yellow urine means your body is dehydrated and has toxic waste to remove. This toxic waste causes your immune system to work overtime in order to keep you healthy. This wasted energy over many years causes you to die decades before your time. This inner toxic waste causes you to age much faster than you ought. Yellow urine is necessary but every trip to the bathroom must not be yellow. When this happens it means you are not drinking enough water.

Your body is just a reflection of an endless cycle of inner planets and universes. The earth is 70 percent water and 30 percent land. Your body is 70 percent plasma and 30 percent membrane. Your cells are 70 percent fluid and 30 percent matter. Are you getting the picture? Yellow urine indicates that your planet is dying of drought and toxic waste. It must be clear at least once a day.

Light Green Urine Color

Light green urine is the result of excess vitamins (i.e. mostly vitamin C) in your urine, causing it to turn a very dark yellow, which may appear green. In your healthful living routine you must overload on vitamins. Take twice-a-day, mega-dose multi vitamins. If you have a problem with iron, then take the vitamins that do not contain iron.

This urine color is healthy and non-toxic to your body. It indicates your body has met its vitamin need and your body is releasing the excess. This makes for very expensive urine, but then you can afford this kind of waste--no pun intended. This eases the amount of chemicals your digestive system has to produce to extract those same vitamins from your food. Your body will still release chemicals to break down the food, but the amounts and types of chemicals are less since you already have a day's supply from the vitamins. Thus, your digestive system secretes fewer chemicals and the workload on your body is reduced.

Drinking Water Promotes Weight Loss and Good Health

Donald S. Robertson, M.D., states:

"Water suppresses the appetite naturally and helps the body metabolize stored fat. Studies have shown that a decrease in water intake will cause fat deposits to increase, while an increase in water intake can actually reduce fat deposits.

Here's Why. The kidneys can't function properly without enough water. When they don't work to capacity, some of their load is dumped onto the liver.

One of the liver's primary functions is to metabolize stored fat into usable energy for the body. But, if the liver has to do some of the kidney's work, it can't operate at full throttle. As a result, it metabolizes less fat, more fat remains stored in the body, and weight loss stops.

Drinking enough water is the best treatment for fluid retention. When the body gets less water, it perceives this as a threat to survival and begins to hold on to every drop. Water is stored in extra-cellular spaces (outside the cells). This shows up as swollen feet, legs, and hands.

Water helps rid the body of waste. During weight loss the body has a lot more waste to get rid of--all that metabolized fat must be shed. Again, adequate water helps flush out the waste.

How much water is enough? On the average, a person needs to drink eight 8 ounce glasses every day. That's about 2 quarts. However, the overweight person needs one additional glass for every 25 pounds of excess weight. The amount you drink may be increased if you exercise briskly or if the weather is hot and dry.

Water must preferably be cold--It's absorbed into the system more quickly than warm water. And some evidence suggests that drinking cold water can actually help burn calories."

Take vitamin suppliments

Take vitamin supplements twice a day to limit gastrointestinal chemical production. The body needs a wide variety of vitamins and minerals for good health. The purpose of a balanced diet is to make certain your body extracts the necessary vitamins and minerals during digestion. If a required vitamin or mineral is deficient in your diet, your body reacts by producing counter chemical reactions that manifest in the form of sickness or disease. An example is vitamin C deficiency, which produces the ailment Scurvy. Likewise, a lack of vitamin D produces the ailment Rickets. Take vitamin supplements twice a day: once before your first meal and once before your last meal. Buy supplements made specifically to take twice a day. Taking vitamins twice a day spreads the dosage over the entire day, further ensuring that your body never runs low and becomes deficient.

Presently, there is a huge debate over whether or not vitamin supplements are necessary if a person eats a balanced diet. Except for the non-water soluble vitamins and minerals (e.g. Iron), any excess is flushed from the system. Therefore, vitamin supplements serve as an insurance policy that, if for some reason you don't ingest via diet all the required vitamins and minerals, your digestion process does not have to produce any counter-chemical reactions.

Before taking any dietary supplement please consult with your physician first. Although vitamin supplements are beneficial when taken correctly, improper usage can lead to medical complications. For example, since iron is not water soluble, excess iron in the body does not flush out and for some people this could lead to a toxic reaction. Also, certain water-soluble vitamins at high dose levels can be toxic to your body (e.g. vitamin A). Therefore, it is important to consult your physician before taking any supplements to ensure that you do not compromise your health.

Eat fewer, smaller, balanced meals

The Food and Drug Administration recommends a balanced diet composed of the 4 basic food groups namely: dairy, meats, vegetables and fruits, and breads and cereals. You must eat less meat, dairy, breads and cereals, and eat more fruits and vegetables.

One key to a longer life is to limit the number of times you eat. As Ben Franklin said, *"to lengthen thy days, lessen thy meals."* By limiting the number of meals for example from three to one, and flushing your system of all impurities with large amounts of water, you reduce the toxic waste production by two-thirds. The Honorable Elijah D. Muhammad documented this concept of eating one meal a day in his best selling book, *Eat To Live*.

Research on Aging reinforces this fact. In a New Jersey Star Ledger newspaper article dated June 1, 1996 titled, *If you eat and be merry, you'll never live to 160*, Dr. George Roth a top scientist at the federal government's National Institute on Aging, citing animal studies said,

"Having less access to food resets the mechanism so that the body can get by with less energy. Furthermore, everything shifts from a growth-and-reproduction strategy to a survival strategy." Make it your goal to reduce the number of times a day you eat. If you are diabetic, pregnant, take prescription medication, or suffer from an eating disorder, then consult your physician before reducing the number of times you eat.

Limit your daily cholesterol to 150mg and reduce your sugar intake

Limit your daily cholesterol intake to 150mg or less per day. A simple method to measure this goal of 150mg is to limit your consumption of meat and dairy products to one serving a day. This inhibits the body from producing low-density lipoprotein--commonly known as bad cholesterol or LDL. Granted, this recommendation is half of what the FDA recommends. Currently 300 mg is recommended. But, this restriction is prudent since the number one killer in America is clogged arteries and veins. Your heart may be under too much stress because you have clogged the arteries and veins with cholesterol. You are literally eating yourself to death.

There are three books on the market that provide several months worth of menu planning to reach the 150mg goal. The first book on dieting for anti-aging purposes is ***Dr. Mollen's Anti-Aging Diet***, written by Dr. Art Mollen. It allows you to eat from the 4 basic food groups, which makes it easy to do. The bottom line of this diet plan is you are allowed to eat one animal protein a day.

The second book is ***Fit for Life***, written by Harvey and Marilyn Diamond. It is one of the all-time, best-selling health and diet books. It is probably the healthiest of diets, but its drawback is you need iron will power to stick to the plan. It has some very strict rules. The bottom line of this diet is to eliminate animal protein and all dairy products from your diet. Fruit must never be eaten with or directly following anything. You must not eat more than one concentrated food at a time--a concentrated food is any food that is not a fruit or a vegetable.

The third book is ***Sugar Busters***, written by H. Leighton Steward, Morrison Bethea, M.D., Sam Andrews, M.D. and Luis Balart, MD. This book is an excellent resource for losing weight and reducing the amount of sugar in your blood. It allows you to eat from the 4 basic food groups, which makes it easy to do. The bottom line of this diet is you must replace the consumption of high-glycemic starches such as, white rice, white bread, white potatoes, carrots, pastas, and corn, with low-glycemic foods such as brown rice, whole wheat bread, sweet potatoes, and green leafy vegetables. Your digestive system converts starches into sugar. The body metabolizes sugar with the hormone insulin. Excess insulin facilitates the storage of fat in fat cells as triglycerides and prevents the breakdown of glycogen and fat in your body. Reducing starch and sugar in your diet reduces the rate of fat storage.

Eat fiber with every meal

You have probably heard the old folks saying *"an apple a day keeps the doctor away."* There is a lot of truth in this saying because it gives the body enough fiber to eliminate much of the waste for one meal. People that ate an apple a day were sick less than the people that didn't. That's how folk tales live.

Fiber acts as a broom in your intestines, sweeping out all the waste. You must eat fiber with each meal. Sure, one apple a day keeps the doctor away; but fiber with each meal keeps old age away. Eating fiber with each meal will sweep away the toxic waste that resides in your digestive system. That waste is one of the reasons you are dying decades before your time. You don't need to eat an apple with each meal but you do need to eat a fiber fruit, fiber vegetable (e.g. lettuce), or dietary fiber supplement with each meal to ensure that your body efficiently removes all the waste from your intestinal system during bowel elimination.

There is a theory of food combining documented in the book *Fit for Life*, which requires you to not combine certain foods for better bowel movements. Fruits when combined with other food types digest slowly and stay in the digestive system longer causing fermentation in the digestive system. Thus, don't combine fruits with other foods. Eat them separately. The important thing is to make sure you have fiber with every meal.

Fiber in your diet is an important part of making elimination more efficient, but fiber does not control when elimination occurs. The process that controls elimination is metabolism.

Exercise before each meal to increase your metabolism

I keep six honest serving men, They taught me all I knew, Their names were When and Where and What, and How and Why and Who." Rudyard Kipling

Metabolism is your body's ability to convert the food you eat into energy and waste products. A large number of people believe their metabolism is set internally and is out of their control, much like a thermometer measures your body temperature. Metabolism is more like a thermostat that can be set to whatever levels you like. Each person does have a biological setting. Some people's metabolism is naturally higher than others. Some people seem to eat and never gain weight, while others seem to gain weight by just walking past a bakery. The good news is your metabolism works like a thermostat and you set the level with exercise. If your metabolism is naturally low, then you must exercise more, which is a blessing in disguise.

Picture in your mind a fireplace with a roaring flame. If you place a big log on that flame, it immediately starts to burn. Yet, if you place that same big log on a fireplace with a small flame, it takes a long time before it burns. Think of your metabolism as a fireplace with a flame set by nature. Some people have a roaring flame, while others have a birthday candle flame. Think of exercise as pouring fuel over the flame. The larger the fire, the quicker things burn. Let us look back at Rudyard Kipling's quotation and answer the questions regarding the when, where, what, how, why and who of exercising for ageless long life.

Why do we need to exercise?

The purpose of exercise is to increase the rate of your body's breathing and blood flow before you eat, in order to more efficiently and effectively transform the food to energy in the form of nutrients and to quickly eliminate any excess waste. The key is to exercise before a meal, which increases the speed at which the waste is created, thereby speeding up the elimination process.

When is the best time to exercise?

Exercising before each meal is a daily minimum requirement in your quest for a 120-year life span. The amount of times you exercise is directly related to the number of times you eat per day. How many times you eat per day refers to large meals like breakfast, lunch and dinner. Light snacks are not included. Don't think you must run laps ever time you want to eat a snack. If you eat three large meals, then you must exercise three times per day. Likewise, if you eat four large meals then you must exercise four times per day.

How do you exercise for long life success?

A good exercise must increase your breathing and blood circulation. Cutting cholesterol in your diet helps the blood flow through your veins. Even if the veins are not clogged with cholesterol you need to ensure minimum travel time for the blood by accelerating the heart muscle during exercise. Deep and heavy breathing with an increased heart rate causes the blood to quickly carry nutrients and oxygen the body needs. The best way to achieve this goal is to do no-impact full-body aerobic exercises

Exercise Aerobically

To do aerobic exercise means exercises that cause you to breath heavily over a long period of time. You may ask, "don't I breathe all the time anyway, so why make such a distinction?" The answer is no. With many exercises you may sometime hold your breath. A good example of holding your breath when exercising is running a sprint race. The runner holds his or her breath for much of the race. This type of exercise is called non-aerobic. Bowling and lifting weights are also non-aerobic activities. Some of the best aerobic exercises are ski-treadmill machines and swimming.

Exercise your entire body

Make sure that when you exercise, every part of your body moves. To qualify as a full-body exercise, you will move both your arms and your legs at the same time. This ensures that every part of your body is in top physical shape versus just one or two parts. Have balance in the exercises you choose. Almost every exercise you do can be incorporated into a full-body routine with a little thought. Some exercises that are already full-body are swimming, skiing, treadmills, and skating.

Exercise with no impact

When you exercise, make sure that there is no impact to your joints. Recall the analogy of your digestive system as a fireplace and exercise as pouring fuel on the flame. The wrong exercises may increase the flame in the sort term, but in the long term wear out the capability to increase that flame due to damaged joints. This is the classic problem of killing the goose that lays the golden egg. The egg represents that benefit you receive from exercise (e.g. lost weight, increased self-esteem). The goose represents the capability to produce that egg in the form of some physical exercise, such as jogging. The person jogs to get the benefit of losing weight. Over time the very exercise causes a problem in the joints, thereby eliminating the method of losing weight and further compromising your health by having joint pain.

A short list of non-impact exercises includes, yoga, stretching, swimming, bicycling, ski treadmills and walking.

What exercises provide long life success?

Listed below are seven beneficial exercises that you can perform before each meal. These exercises have the benefits of being non-impact, aerobic, total body, and fun.

Total body stretching or yoga every day

Stretching is something you must do before and after you exercise. Stretching ensures that your body is flexible and prevents injuries. Make sure that you do full-body stretching. To begin your stretching exercises start from the top of your head and stretch every part of your body working down to the bottom of your feet:

1. Stretch your face muscles.
2. Stretch your neck muscles.
3. Stretch your shoulder muscles.
4. Stretch your arm muscles.
5. Stretch your wrist.
6. Stretch your hands.
7. Stretch your fingers by doing finger tip pushups.
8. Stretch your chest/ breast muscles.
9. Stretch your stomach muscles.
10. Stretch your back muscles.
11. Stretch your buttock muscles.
12. Stretch your knees by rotating them in a circle.
13. Stretch your thigh muscles.
14. Stretch your ankles.
15. Stretch your calf.
16. Stretch your feet.
17. Stretch your toes.

Yoga incorporates deep breathing as part of your stretching. You are not fully living your potential life span, and one reason is you are only using 50% or less of your lung's breathing capacity. The more fresh air that you can deliver to the blood; the better you metabolize everything you ingested.

Sit quietly for a moment and breathe in through your nose and try to fill your lungs as full as they can get without exploding. Exhale very slowly through your mouth. Specific yoga exercises are described in detail in the first chapter.

Swimming

Swimming is an excellent exercise you can do that is a full-body, no-impact, and aerobic activity. Swim at least once every other week.

Try to work up to swimming 1600 meters (a little over a mile). That is 32 laps in a 25-meter pool. When you first start swimming, one lap may be very hard to do. Every day swim a little bit farther, and before you know it you are swimming a mile.

No impact full-body treadmill machines

A treadmill machine is one of the best exercises you can do because it is a full-body, no-impact, and aerobic activity. Make sure the machine moves both the arms and legs at the same time. Do this at least 3 times a week. This is a piece of equipment you may consider purchasing for your home. It provides an alternative indoor workout when the weather outside is inclement.

Walking

Walking is another wonderful exercise to do because it is a full-body, non-impact, and aerobic activity. Do this at least 3 times a week. Do this exercise during lunchtime if you work. It is a convenient exercise that does not require a shower afterward.

Rollerblading or Ice Skating

Skating on wheels or ice is a fun exercise that is a full-body, non-impact, and aerobic activity. Do this at least 3 times a week. These exercises are also particularly good since they are fun and popular. If you are a beginning skater take lessons to reduce the likelihood of injury and wear protective clothing and equipment.

Total body weight lifting twice a week

Lifting slows the aging process by strengthening the muscles that support the bones and skin that with age usually weaken and cause the body to deteriorate much faster than necessary. *"Lifting strengthens the bones by taking off the load of work necessary for the bones to support the body over time."* This statement was made by Doug Levy in a December 1994 USA Today, headline *Pumping Iron Helps Bones of Older Women*.

"Pumping iron twice a week can sharply reduce risk of osteoporosis and resulting broken bones among older women," says a study in today's Journal of the American Medical Association.

"A 45-minute workout using five different weight lifting machines twice a week has more benefits than estrogen-replacement therapy or other treatments to prevent osteoporosis," says leading author Miriam Nelson of Tufts University, Boston. The study followed 39 women ages 50-70 who were not on estrogen therapy or other medications affecting bone density. The 20 women who did weight training had 1% more density at the end of the year-long study. The 19 who did not train lost 2.5% of their bone density. The iron-pumping group also had improved balance and muscle strength. "I would say we turned the clock back 15 to 20 years," says Nelson.

The problem with many weight lifting programs is they are not full-body. Many programs neglect the very parts of your bodies that age the fastest. With this in mind, you need to focus on those neglected areas. Arnold Schwarzenegger wrote a good book on the subject that is easy to read and exercises the entire body. The book is entitled, **Arnold: The Education of a Bodybuilder.** It is his autobiography as a bodybuilder. The last chapter of the book provides an excellent weight lifting program suitable for any person who wants to begin.

Play a lifetime resort sport once a week

Find an active lifetime resort sport to occupy your free time. The most popular resort sports are golf, tennis, scuba diving and snorkeling. These activities are extremely popular sports throughout the world. Whenever you take vacations, they can become mini sports adventures. Almost every resort in the world provides these activities so you can exercise while you travel and vacation. These are also sports that you can do at any age.

Where are places to organize your exercise routine?

There are three places to organize your exercise routine around that allows you to exercise before every meal: your home, your job, and your health club.

At home

A large amount of your exercise program will occur at home. You have many options to choose from, like home workout videos, exercise equipment for your home gym and exercises that originate from your home--jogging, walking and biking. Exercising immediately after waking up is the most convenient way to ensure you get your workout done.

At work

If you are lucky your job may have exercise facilities on site, or you may work close enough to a health club you can visit during your lunch break. If you are not lucky enough to have the first two options you still have the ultimate lunchtime exercise--walking. The key is to take a nice brisk walk before you eat lunch. Walk for a minimum of 30 minutes at a brisk pace. This still gives you another 30 to 15 minutes to eat lunch. On days when the weather is bad outside climb stairs while swinging your arms (assuming you have some stairs to climb). Even if there are only a few flights, just walk up and down for 30 minutes. You will get a good workout and prime your metabolism.

At a health club

Join a health club that has the following features: a swimming pool large enough for you to swim laps, a large number of full-body treadmill machines, weight lifting equipment, and aerobics classes with trained instructors.

Your health club membership is just as valuable as your medical insurance for maintaining health. Where you spend your money is a good indication of what you believe is important. A fully utilized health club membership prevents many of the health problems your health insurance pays to resolve.

Who do you exercise with for long life success?

Pick a buddy that motivates you to workout. You need someone who can share the load. There will be times when you won't want to exercise and your buddy will be there to help you. Your first choice for a buddy must be your mate. This longevity program requires a significant amount of time and exercising together is a good social outlet that you can share. If you have children, this is an excellent outlet to facilitate family bonding.

A sample 7-day program that combines exercise and diet

Until you coordinate your eating habits with your exercise habits, you will continue to age faster--and ultimately live a shorter life--since your body is constantly under the stress of processing toxic waste. The average American diet consists of about three large meals per day. That means the average American needs to exercise three times a day. This may seem overwhelming at first, but listed below is a sample 7-day program by which this can easily be accomplished. The meals in this example limit your daily cholesterol to less than 150mg without sacrificing your enjoyment for eating delicious food. You will drink one gallon of water each day. The exercises before the meals allows you to eliminate the toxic waste from your system as quickly as possible; and drinking large amounts of water and taking vitamins allows you to urinate in three different colors during the day. This 7-day program puts into practice all the habits you have just learned.

Day 1

Breakfast

Workout: Drink ½ quart of water before and after the workout. Ride for 30 minutes on a stationary bike at a brisk pace. Then stretch for flexibility and do 25 sit-ups, 25 pushups, yoga, prayer, or meditation for 10 minutes.

Food: Take a multi-vitamin and wash it down with 1 quart of water before eating your breakfast. Your meal consists of a banana and an apple. Men should finish their meal by drinking 12-ounce glass of fresh fruit juice. Women should finish their meal by drinking a 12-ounce glass of skim milk or eating an 8-ounce cup of yogurt to get your calcium.

Lunch:

Workout: Drink ½ quart of water before your workout. Do a 20-minute walk at a brisk pace on a flat surface, and then stretch for flexibility.

Food: Drink ½ quart of water before your meal. The meal consists of soup and salad, followed by drinking a 12-ounce glass of 100% fruit juice.

Dinner

Workout: Drink ½ quart of water before your workout. Jog 1/2-mile for warm-up, stretch for flexibility, lift weights for upper-body for 45 minutes, and do 50 sit-ups.

Food: Take a multiple vitamin and wash it down with ½ quart of water before your meal. Your meal consists of fruit juice, salad, vegetarian lasagna, and a bowl of no-fat frozen yogurt for desert.

Day 2

Breakfast

Workout: Drink ½ quart of water before and after the workout. Step for 30 minutes at a brisk pace, on a step machine simultaneously swinging your arm. Then stretch for flexibility and do 25 sit-ups, 25 pushups, yoga, prayer, or meditation for 10 minutes.

Food: Take a multi-vitamin and wash it down with 1 quart of water before eating your breakfast. Your meal consists of a peach and a plum. Men finish you meal by drinking 12-ounce glass of fresh fruit juice. Women should finish their meal by drinking a 12-ounce glass of skim milk or eating an 8-ounce cup of yogurt to get your calcium.

Lunch:

Workout: Drink ½ quart of water before your workout. Walk for 20-minutes at a brisk pace on a flat surface then stretch for flexibility.

Food: Drink ½ quart of water before your meal. The meal consists of soup and a tuna fish sandwich with lettuce and tomato on wheat bread, followed by drinking a 12-ounce glass of 100% fruit juice.

Dinner

Workout: Drink ½ quart of water before your workout. Jog ½-mile to warm-up, and then stretch for flexibility. Go to your martial arts or aerobics class and do 60 sit-ups.

Food: Take a multiple vitamin and wash it down with ½ quart of water before your meal. The meal consists of salad, skinless chicken breast, and baked sweet potato with margarine.

Day 3

Breakfast

Workout: Drink ½ quart of water before and after the workout. Row for 30-minutes at a brisk pace, on a rowing machine. Then stretch for flexibility and do 25 sit-ups, 25 pushups, yoga, prayer, or meditation for 10 minutes.

Food: Take a multi-vitamin and wash it down with 1 quart of water before eating your breakfast. Your meal consists of a banana and sliced cantaloupe. Men should finish their meal by drinking 12-ounce glass of fresh fruit juice. Women should finish their meal by drinking a 12-ounce glass of skim milk or eating an 8-ounce cup of yogurt to get your calcium.

Lunch:

Workout: Drink ½ quart of water before your workout. Walk for 20-minutes at a brisk pace on a flat surface then stretch for flexibility.

Food: Drink ½ quart of water before your meal. The meal consists of a salad with tomatoes, topped with low-fat dressing and pasta covered with a meatless tomato sauce, followed by drinking a 12-ounce glass of 100% fruit juice.

Dinner

Workout: Drink ½ quart of water before your workout. Jog ½ mile to warm up and then stretch for flexibility. Swim as many laps as you can up to 1600 meters.

Food: Take a multiple vitamin and wash it down with ½ quart of water before your meal. Your meal consists of baked flounder over brown rice with steamed broccoli tips, and sorbet for desert

Day 4

Breakfast

Workout: Drink ½ quart of water before and after the workout. Ride for 30 minutes on a stationary bike at a brisk pace. Then stretch for flexibility and do 25 sit-ups, 25 pushups, yoga, prayer, or meditation for 10 minutes.

Food: Take a multi-vitamin and wash it down with 1 quart of water before eating your breakfast. Your meal consists of a banana and 20 cherries. Men should finish their meal by drinking 12-ounce glass of fresh fruit juice. Women should finish their meal by drinking a 12-ounce glass of skim milk or eating an 8-ounce cup of yogurt to get your calcium.

Lunch:

Workout: Drink ½ quart of water before your workout. Walk for 20-minutes at a brisk pace on a flat surface, then stretch for flexibility.

Food: Drink ½ quart of water before your meal. The meal consists of a soup and salad, followed by drinking a 12-ounce glass of 100% fruit juice.

Dinner

Workout: Drink ½ quart of water before your workout. Jog for ½-mile to warm-up and stretch for stretch for flexibility, martial arts or a low-impact aerobic dance for 45 minutes, sit-ups.

Food: Take a multiple vitamin and wash it down with ½ quart of water before your meal. Your meal consists of a salad, skinless turkey breast, cranberries, stuffing, low-fat gravy, and a bowl of no-fat frozen yogurt.

Day 5

Breakfast

Workout: Drink ½ quart of water before and after the workout. Step for 30 minutes at a brisk pace, on a step machine simultaneously swinging your arms. Then stretch for flexibility and do 25 sit-ups, 25 pushups. Then do yoga, prayer, or meditation for 10 minutes.

Food: Take a multi-vitamin and wash it down with 1 quart of water before eating your breakfast. Your meal consists of a banana and fresh sliced pineapple. Men should finish their meal by drinking 12-ounce glass of fresh fruit juice. Women should finish their meal by drinking a 12-ounce glass of skim milk or eating an 8-ounce cup of yogurt to get your calcium.

Lunch:

Workout: Drink ½ quart of water before your workout. Walk for 20-minutes at a brisk pace on a flat surface then stretch for flexibility.

Food: Drink ½ quart of water before your meal. The meal consists of a grilled chicken sandwich with lettuce and tomato on wheat bread and a side of mixed vegetables, followed by drinking a 12-ounce glass of 100% fruit juice.

Dinner

Workout: Drink ½ quart of water before your workout. Jog for ½-mile to warm-up and stretch for stretch for flexibility, lift weights for lower-body for 45 minutes, and do 25 push-ups.

Food: Take a multiple vitamin and wash it down with ½ quart of water before your meal. Your meal consists of shrimp scampi served over brown rice, mixed vegetables, and a slice of cherry pie.

Day 6

Breakfast

Workout: Drink ½ quart of water before and after the workout. Play a social recreation sport (e.g. golf, tennis, bowling).

Food: Take a multi-vitamin and wash it down with 1 quart of water before eating your breakfast. Your meal consists of a banana and 20 strawberries. Men should finish their meal by drinking 12-ounce glass of fresh fruit juice. Women should finish their meal by drinking a 12-ounce glass of skim milk or eating an 8-ounce cup of yogurt to get your calcium.

Lunch:

Workout: Drink ½ quart of water before your workout. Play a social recreation sport (e.g. golf, tennis, bowling).

Food: Drink ½ quart of water before your meal. The meal consists of a grilled chicken Cesar salad topped with low-fat Cesar dressing, followed by drinking a 12-ounce glass of 100% fruit juice.

Dinner

Workout: Jog ½-mile for warm-up, stretch for flexibility. Play a social recreation sport (e.g. golf, tennis, bowling).

Food: Take a multiple vitamin and wash it down with ½ quart of water before your meal. Your meal consists of a salad, rotisserie chicken, and low-fat gravy, cream spinach, and no-fat yogurt covered with raisins.

Day 7

Breakfast

Workout: Drink ½ quart of water before and after the workout. Do yoga, prayer, or meditation for 10 minutes.

Food: Take a multi-vitamin and wash it down with 1 quart of water before eating your breakfast. Your meal consists of a nectarine and a tangerine. Men should finish their meal by drinking 12-ounce glass of fresh fruit juice. Women should finish their meal by drinking a

12-ounce glass of skim milk or eating an 8-ounce cup of yogurt to get your calcium.

Lunch:

Workout: Do yoga, prayer, or meditation for 10 minutes.

Food: Drink ½ quart of water before your meal. The meal consists of a grilled tuna steak or salmon steak sandwich with lettuce and tomato on wheat bread and a side of mixed vegetables, followed by drinking a 12-ounce glass of 100% fruit juice.

Dinner

Workout: Do yoga, prayer, or meditation for 10 minutes.

Food: Take a multiple vitamin and wash it down with ½ quart of water before your meal. Your meal consists of Oriental stir-fry vegetables in garlic sauce over brown rice, and graham crackers and skim milk for desert.

Monitor your blood pressure, your cholesterol and your weight

There are three numbers that you must know which affect your health:

- Your blood pressure
- Your blood cholesterol
- Your weight

The leading killers today are heart disease, stroke, and diabetes, which are all related to your blood and obesity. These diseases are contracted primarily by your habits of nutrition and exercise. Knowing your blood numbers and weight is a good indication of how well you are doing on the quest to live 120 years in outstanding health. If your numbers are not optimal then you are at risk of not reaching this goal. Blood pressure and cholesterol tests have been scientifically proven to accurately predict your level of risk. The health habits you have just learned can provide you with excellent numbers.

Every other year get a complete physical examination from a board certified doctor that practices internal medicine. Included in the exam are blood tests that measure your cholesterol and pressure levels. Your doctor may tell you to factor in your age as it applies to your cholesterol, pressure, and weight. If you are older, then your numbers can be less than optimal. With the comforting words, "these results are good for a person your age"; you are being lulled to an early grave. To live 120 years in excellent health your goal is to have optimal numbers no matter what your age.

Your blood cholesterol goal must be less than 200 for your total cholesterol count, less than 130 for your LDL count, and greater than 60 for your HDL count. If any of these numbers are significantly out of range then you are at risk for heart disease. Cholesterol is an essential nutrient produced naturally in your body for repairing cell membranes and producing hormones. But when you consume too much cholesterol by eating saturated fats, the excess cholesterol your body does not use is deposited on the lining of your veins and arteries. Over time this buildup restricts the flow of blood, contributing to high blood pressure and depriving vital tissues in your heart of the blood-borne oxygen they need. This contributes to serious damage called arteriosclerosis.

Your blood pressure numbers must be less than or equal to 130/85. The 130 represent the systolic pressure, which is the pressure of the blood going through your veins when the heart is contracted. The 85 represent the diastolic pressure, which is the pressure of the blood going through your veins when the heart is at rest. If your numbers are above 140/90 then you need to lower them at once.

People who are overweight or obese have a greater chance of getting high blood pressure, high cholesterol and diabetes. Therefore, it is important to measure your weight to ensure you are not overweight or obese. The Body Mass Index (BMI) is an index of a person's weight in relation to height. A BMI score of 18.5 to 24.9 indicates a healthy body fat ratio. A BMI score of 25.0 or more indicates an individual is overweight. A BMI score of 30 or more indicates an individual is obese.

If you have access to the Internet, then former Surgeon General, Dr. C. Everett Koop has an excellent website with a BMI calculator that is very easy to use. The web address is ***http://drkoop.com.*** If you don't have Internet access then calculate it on your own. Just multiply your weight by 703 and divide the result by your height in inches--squared. For example if a person is 6'3" tall and weights 194 pounds the calculation for BMI is as follows: (194 x 703) / (75 x 75) = 136382 / 5625 = 24.2.

BMI values apply to both men and women, regardless of their age, frame size, or muscle mass. These values do not apply to athletes and body builders, pregnant and nursing women, frail or elderly persons or persons under 18.

You have learned exercise and nutrition habits that can produce superior blood test results. For some people these numbers do not get on track utilizing these natural methods. If your numbers are bad, then you need to consider other alternatives such as herbs and pharmaceutical drugs. For lowering your blood pressure with herbs, the book, *Prescription for Nutritional Healing* states,

> "Cayenne (capsicum), chamomile, fennel, hawthorn berries, parsley, and rosemary. Caution: Do not use chamomile on an ongoing basis, as ragweed allergy may result. Avoid it completely if you are allergic to ragweed. Avoid the herbs ephedra (ma hung) and ticorice, as these herbs can elevate blood pressure."

If you choose to use pharmaceutical drugs to lower your blood pressure there are several angiotensin converting enzyme inhibitor drugs on the market. Two drugs you might consider are Monopril and Captopril. These drugs have been effective in lower blood pressure and thus extending life.

For lowering your blood cholesterol with herbs, the book, *Prescription for Nutritional Healing* states,

> "Cayenne, goldenseal, and hawthorn berries. Also Spirulina taken on a daily basis. Caution: Do not take goldenseal internally on a daily basis for more than one week at a time. Do not use it during pregnancy and use it with caution if you are allergic to ragweed."

If you choose to use pharmaceutical drugs to lower your blood cholesterol there is a lipid-lowering drug know as Pravastatin. This drug has been approved for use in healthy people with elevated cholesterol to prevent the first heart attack and reduce the risk of death.

Bibliography for the 5th Principle

1. Ancient Secret of the Fountain of Youth, Peter Kelder, Doubleday
2. Dr. Mollen's Anti-Aging Diet, Art Mollen, Dutton Publishing
3. Drink Water to Keep The Fat Away, Donald S. Robertson, M.D., M. Sc.
4. Earl Mindells Vitamin Bible, Earl Mindell, Warner Books
5. Eat Right For your Type: The Individualized Diet Solution to Staying Healthy, Living Longer, & Achieving Your Ideal Weight, Dr. Peter J. D'Adamo, Putnam Press
6. Eat to Win, Dr. Robert Hass, Signet Publishing
7. Eight Weeks to Optimum Health, Andrew Weil, Fawcett Book Group
8. Fit for Life, Harvey and Marilyn Diamond, Warner Books Inc.
9. Healing with Vitamins, Editors of Prevention Magazine, Rodale
10. How to Eat to Live, The Hon. Elijah D. Muhammad, Propagation Society
11. Life Extension: A Practical Scientific Approach, D. Pearson & S. Shaw, Warner Books
12. Nutrition Action Health Letter, 1875 Connecticut Ave. N.W., Suite 300, Washington, DC 20009-5728 (202) 332-9110
13. Perscription for Nutritional Healing, Phyllis Balch, CNC and James F. Balch MD, Avery Press
14. Personal Trainer Manual: The Resource for Fitness Instructors, American Council on Exercise, Reebok University Press
15. Snowbird Diet, Donald S. Robertson, Carol P. Robertson, Warner Books, Incorporated
16. Sugar Busters, H. Leighton Steward, Morrison Bethea, M.D., Sam Andrews, M.D. and Luis Balart, MD, Harper Audio
17. The Education of a Bodybuilder, Arnold Schwarzenegger with Douglas Kent Hall, Simon & Schuster
18. The Zone, Barry Sears, HarperCollins
19. Your Body's Many Cries for Water, F. Batmonghelidj, MD, Global Health Solutions, Incorporated

Refuse to age gracefully

This principle may not be for you. Some people say that they enjoy looking older, looking more mature with time. They are proud of their gray or silver hair; it is their badge of distinction. They honor their wrinkles, for they show the character of a well-spent life. They don't mind looking older, they just want to feel energetic and age in a healthy and graceful way. This is a wonderful point of view.

If you practice every other principle in this book but skip this principle and you don't mind looking old, you may still live 120 years in good health. The only problem is when you are 120 years you will look 90 years old. If you read and practice the methods discussed in this principle, you may live 120 years but never look older than 50. The choice is yours.

Theory: The human body ages slower when a good maintence plan is followed, which affects the self image and the eventual will to live.

Imagine for a moment that you live on a planet were the human spirit resides inside a car instead of skin, flesh and bones. Some people are born Corvettes, some Pintos, some Chevy vans, etc. The average life span for a car is about 200,000 miles. There are some cars on this planet that seem to never age regardless of how many miles they have. They have been labeled by society as restored antiques. A 57 Chevy, a 67 Mustang, a 56 Corvette, all look today just like when they were first born. Other cars have plenty of excuses to explain why these restored antiques look so good for their age. Some of the excuses you have heard or even said yourself such as, they're lucky; they have rich owners who can afford to keep them up; they're vain, and they have good genes.

Let's return to the real planet Earth for a moment. You will be presented with examples throughout this chapter with this car metaphor in mind. The goal is for you to become a restored antique. There is no reason you have to look older than you want to once you reach your middle-to-late twenties. Some people take good care of their cars, some take outstanding care, and some take lousy care. The majority of people just do what they are told. You must determine the level of care you are going to take for your body, whether it is covered with flesh or auto parts.

The car metaphor is easy to understand since many people treat their cars and their houses better than they treat themselves. Not everyone owns a house, but almost everyone at some time in his or her life owns a car. You drive your car down the highway called life. If you understand this car metaphor, you understand a large part of this teaching. You choose the appearance of your car, and although car styles change from year to year, nothing on your car has to look old unless you let it. If parts wear out, replace them. If something breaks, fix it. The key to keeping your car looking and running like new is to always attend to the maintenance of the little things before they become big things.

There is pressure in this world to get rid of your old car and buy a new one, "don't chase good money after bad." This is the same kind of peer pressure that allows your flesh and bones body to prematurely appear older. There is definite peer pressure to wear out your body and age just like everyone else.

You don't just wake up one Sunday morning, look in the mirror and say, "Gee, I look 20 years older today!" The aging of your looks is a gradual process, which takes place on a daily basis with the "little things." We are going to explore a philosophy of grooming that eliminates those little things on a daily basis so that your looks stay consistent over time.

Fight natural aging and keep your body looking new

If you look old and feel tired and weak, you won't take the time and effort to treat yourself as good as you would if you looked young and felt healthy and strong. The reason you won't is because of the **Psychology of Accelerated Depreciation**. This principle is exemplified in how you care for a new car and stop caring once it gets old.

When you buy a new car, you may at first give it an inordinate amount of attention. As it gets older and you are ready for another new car, you might fail to give it the necessary attention that would keep it on the road running good. You eventually kill your car to justify buying a new one. This same principle holds true with your body. Eliminating the appearance of age indicators such as gray hair, wrinkles, high blood pressure and high cholesterol is not for vain reasons; it's to counteract the psychology of accelerated depreciation. The more of these little indicators you see and feel, the easier it is to grow old and die decades before your time. Since society is content for you to die at 80, it tells you to not worry about these little things, as that's how God intended it to be. At some point, your mind decides you have had enough pain and suffering and you welcome death.

Practice positive self-talk when looking in the mirror

How you talk to yourself in the mirror each day as you groom yourself is important for ageless long life. Like Narcissus, you must fall in love with your reflection. If you don't love yourself, then who will? Beauty is a subjective concept and you are entitled to your opinion.

Try this experiment for the next week. Wake up and take a good look at yourself in the mirror. Notice every blemish, hair, and pore on your skin. When you wake up the next day do the same exercise and look for differences. How much you have aged in that 24-hour period? Your answer is obvious; nothing has changed. The reason you do not see any differences is due to cognitive dissonance in your ability to perceive change. In other words, your mind masks minor changes from your perceptions. That is why you can go away for the summer, gain 30 pounds and not really notice the change; but when you return, all your friends notice the difference immediately.

Therefore, take periodic pictures of your body in just a swimming suit and compare the pictures on a semi-annual basis. This method moves your conscious mind from the role of subjective observer into the role of objective observer.

While looking at yourself in the mirror during grooming, memorize the following affirmation by Louise L. Hay from her book, *You Can Heal Your Life* and say it to out loud every day for the rest of our life:

"In the infinity of where I am, all is perfect, whole, and complete. I recognize my body as a good friend. Each cell in my body has divine intelligence. I listen to what it tells me, and I know its advice is valid. I am always safe, and Divinely protected and guided. I choose to be healthy and free. All is well in my world."

Your appearance is a reflection of light

Your appearance is in many ways an illusion. The real you is divine, eternal and pure energy. You are a child of light. Your light essence lives in a planet, which requires a body. That body is not you; it is just a reflection of a body you temporally inhabit, seen through eyes that depend on light for vision. The absence or increase of light significantly alters your appearance to others. For example, the models you see in the magazines are under light so intense that their skin appears flawless to the sight.

Anything that alters your reflection from the light alters your appearance and causes you to look older. Think about a baby fresh from the mother's womb. It has pure skin and a flawless complexion. As that child grows its skin changes and things start to grow on it such as hair, freckles, moles, and warts. All of these changes reflect the light and cause that person to appear older. Therefore, the crux of the philosophy of ageless grooming is to keep your skin as free from alteration as possible.

Eliminate the indicators of age before they take root

In a society obsessed with appearance and youth, the ability to determine a person's age is still very subjective. For example, there was a museum guide who gave a tour of the dinosaurs at a Jurassic park and told the crowd that the skeleton of the Brontosaurus was 5,000,023 years old. One of the children asked how he was so certain of the exact age. The guide said, "I was told it was 5 million years old when I started working here 23 years ago."

You guess at a person's age based on subjective visual indicators. No one has ever taught you how to do this. It is an intuitive skill you learn throughout life. There are 26 significant indicators that people use to guess your age. The more of them you have, the older you appear.

Surprisingly, there are solutions to reduce or eliminate the appearance of all 26 indicators. Listed below are the indicators:

1. Sun damaged skin
2. Wrinkles
3. Uneven skin tone
4. Excessive and poorly groomed body hair
5. Shaving bumps
6. Moles
7. Age spots and liver spots
8. Varicose veins
9. Acute facial lines
10. Sagging neck skin
11. Eye glasses
12. Bags underneath the eyes
13. Eye lenses that are not white
14. Crows feet in the corners of the eyes
15. Smoker's face
16. Visible dental work
17. Discolored teeth
18. Gray hair
19. Balding or thinning hair
20. Hair protruding from the ear
21. Hair protruding from the nose
22. Un-groomed eyebrows
23. Corns and bunions on the feet
24. Old sounding voice
25. Excessive weight
26. Poor posture

There was a time when these indicators of aging would give away your age. Advances in medicine, nutrition, cosmetic surgery, and physical fitness have made it possible to remove or significantly reduce the appearance of almost every indicator of aging. Without these indicators it is extremely difficult for any person to know your age unless you decide to tell them. There are three methods to eliminate or reduce the appearance of age indicators: exercise, surgery, and covering them up. In the sections that follow, each indicator is discussed and alternatives provided on how to reduce or eliminate them.

Many of the methods to eliminate or reduce these indicators require hard work. Many of the remedies in this section are not new, earth shattering, or complex; they are common sense but not common knowledge. Many are methods of grooming that for some reason are not a part of the human process of acceptability. Make these grooming habits the norm and not the exception in your grooming routine. Let's examine how to eliminate or reduce the majority of these indicators.

Remove any growth and replace any loss that reflects age

In order for you to get the most out of this program you may have to change your beliefs about the topic of cosmetic surgery. Although public attitude is changing, it still carries a stigma. Many times we see the supermarket tabloids blasting the latest celebrity that altered her nose or breasts. In general, surgery is a scary subject. Many people have surgery to correct problems with their health. So, some perceive the idea of subjecting yourself to pain for cosmetic reasons as vain and self-centered.

There is nothing "plastic" about surgery. The word plastic has a very negative connotation that is synonymous with phony or shallow. Originally, plastic surgery derived its name from the time when the procedures dealt primarily with the reshaping of bones, and skin. You must begin to remove any stigma associated with cutting one part of the body over another and accept that your psychological health is just as important as your physical health.

The medical definition of surgery is the cutting, removing, or reconstructing of the human body in order to improve health. If you agree with this definition, then you perform surgery on yourself on a weekly or even a daily basis. Here are some surgeries you perform on your body:

- Going to the beauty salon or barber to cut your hair
- Clipping your toenails and fingernails when they get too long.
- Shaving

All of these are acts of surgery that you do on a daily or weekly basis. They improve either your physical health (dental hygiene) or mental health (positive self-image). What makes your hair anymore important than your nose or your breasts? Remember the definition of surgery it to cut to improve your health. Your self-image has a direct relationship to your physical health. If you cut your hair because it makes you feel better, you have just as much right to cut any other part of your body, if it makes you feel better about yourself. You are cautioned to only do this if your appearance bothers you; never do it to gain social acceptance.

Zig Ziglar, the motivational speaker, in his audio classic, *Success and the Self Image* tells the story of how his daughter although beautiful, intelligent, and happy was not satisfied with the size of her ears. She would always wear hairstyles and hats to cover them up. She did not like the way they stuck out. She was unhappy about her appearance and let her father know about it. He let her have surgery to give her ears the appearance she wanted. She became very happy with the results. The important thing to remember is this is your body and you have the right to be happy with its appearance.

Practice daily grooming of every part of your body

In the area of grooming, society has developed a "pick and choose" attitude as to what constitutes proper grooming. People take immaculate care of one part of their face and yet literally never groom others. For example, when was the last time you ever saw a man groom his eyebrows? A man spends $15 twice a month on haircuts and never takes the time to groom the hair above his eyes. Eyebrows that are not groomed make you look old. This hair is all out of control and bushy. This is an example of "pick and choose" grooming.

Get rid of your pick and choose mentality towards grooming. By following these suggestions, your looks will literally remain constant over decades simply because you are dealing with them in the present moment. Keep this up day in and day out and over time you appear to age slower since your appearance remains consistent and you are practicing a habit that very few people ever do.

Adults must groom differently from children

"When I was a child, I spoke, thought, and reasoned as a child does. But when I became an adult I put away childish things." I Cor 13:11

Each year you must adjust your grooming ritual to meet your current needs. This has been true since the day you were born. Every year you had to learn how to take care of something else on your body to keep yourself clean and presentable. When you reach 18 years of age, you think that you have learned all you need to know about grooming, and for the next sixty years you groom your body in the same manner you did when you were 18. Anything else added to the process is somehow vain, unnatural, or unnecessary. This is yet another attitude you must shed.

Eliminate the unnatural grooming myth

Some types of grooming feel unnatural because they go against nature. For example, coloring gray hair might seem unnatural since nature gave us the gray hair. Much of life is learning to do what is unnatural and making it natural. As Dr. Scott M. Peck states in the book *The Road Less Traveled*,

> "It is also natural to defecate in our pants and never bursh our teeth. Yet we teach ourselves to do the unnatural until the unnatural becomes itself second nature. Indeed all self-discipline might be defined as teaching ourselves to do the unnatural. Another characteristic of human nature--perhaps the one that makes us most human-- is our capacity to do the unnatural, to transend and hence transform our own nature."

Unlike all the other animals that roam the earth, human beings have the ability to reason, change our surroundings, and to change the effects of nature.

Ageless face

> *By the time a person is 40 they have the face they deserve.--Yogi Berra*

Your face is the easiest body part to mold. It reflects your values and beliefs at any given time. Want to see what a person believes? Just look at his or her face. You choose how you want your face to look and you will learn how to keep it looking young, instead of trading it in for an older model.

Don't Buy A Smoker's Face

Of all the bad habits that age your appearance, there is none that compares with smoking. In fact, the aging related to smoking has its own appearance, which is common among all smokers. A person who smokes for over 15 years will have a smoker's face. Below is a picture of the typical smoker's face in old age.

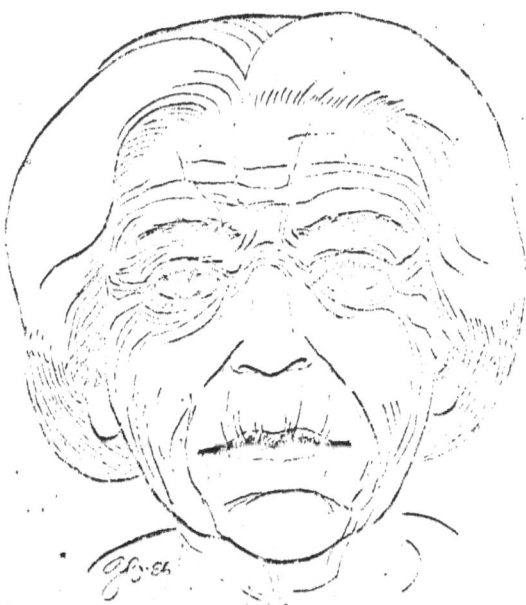

Figure 27—Typical Smokers Face in Old Age

The reason that a smoker's face will quickly age is the result of smoke that lingers on the face just like it lingers on your clothing. Ever go to a bar or social place where smoking is allowed and come home smelling like a cigarette? Well just imagine how much of that smoke is lodged on the smokers face. You just smell the "second hand" smoke that traveled in the air and landed on your clothing. This smoke forms a cloud of dust that eats away at the smoker's skin. This dust contains toxic byproducts such as carbon monoxide, which causes their immune system cells to fight off the penetration of this smoke into their system. This is what over time gives a smoker's skin the appearance of old worn leather. Instead of the top layer of the skin being fresh and new, it is constantly covered with soot and fighting off the toxic chemicals from the layer of smoke.

Another reason that a smoker's face ages faster is the heat damage produced by the cigarette upon the lips and teeth. The heat of a cigarette is hot enough to cook food. Although this flame is a couple inches away from your face, the heat sucked in from the cigarette smoke is still hot enough to cause heat damage to your lips and inside your mouth. Your body was not built to withstand this kind of heat.

Smoking is one of the hardest habits in the world to break, because it provides a natural relaxation sedative from the drug nicotine--and nicotine is addictive. The good news is that public pressure is turning against smoking. No person wants to be looked down upon; many people are succumbing to the pressure and quitting. By the middle of the 21st century peer pressure against smoking will be so vocal that hopefully no one will want to do it anymore.

Don't touch your face

Touching your face with your hand damages your skin. For the next week, just notice how many time a day you put your hands on your face. All this friction adds up and causes your face to look older than necessary. Many teenagers, during puberty, develop the habit of squeezing their pimples, causing scars and developing a bad habit that may last a lifetime. If you have to squeeze your pimples, use 2 cotton swabs instead of your fingers.

Many people sit and read with their hands holding their face to keep the head up. Others put their hands on their face when they are confused or astonished. Whatever particular habits you have developed, it is now time to change them and never touch your face except to clean it and make it look good. This is a habit that takes time and your full awareness to conquer. It may help to ask your friends to tell you just when you are touching it, since many times you do it unconscious.

Exercise your face muscles

Some, but not all of the wrinkles that appear on your face can be removed by exercising your face muscles. Unfortunately, the muscle fiber in the face is not thick enough to counteract all face wrinkles by expanding the muscle density. You will now learn 3 facial exercises to remove some wrinkles and keep your facial skin taunt and youthful.

Take your lips and pucker them like you are going to give someone a kiss. Stretch and push them out as far as possible and hold it there for 10 seconds. You will feel the skin of your lower face get tighter. Do this until your face gets tired. Start slowly, with about 3 sets of 5 repetitions.

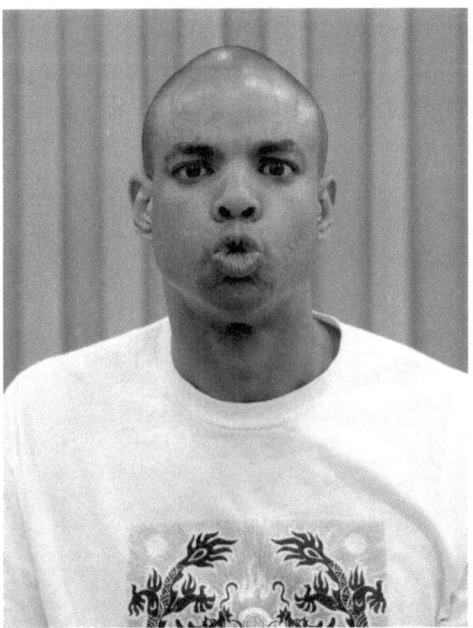

Figure 28—Starting position for Lip Puckers
to firm up the skin around the mouth

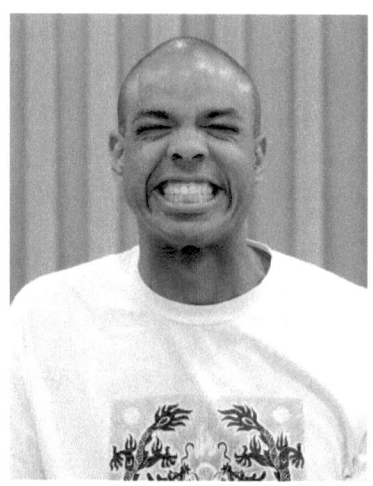

Figure 29—Ending position for Lip Puckers
to firm up the skin around the mouth

Then open your mouth as wide as possible until you feel like your jawbone is going to break. Then form an open circle with your lips and try to move the right side of your mouth to the left as far as possible with your lips and hold it for 10 seconds. Then repeat going from left to right. You will feel the skin under your eye and beside your nose getting tighter. Do this until your face gets tired. Start slowly, with about 3 sets of 5 repetitions.

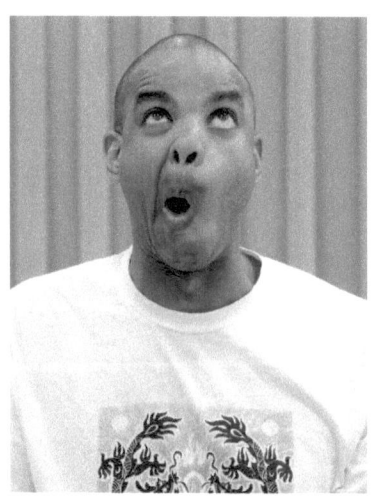

Figure 30—Starting position for Cheek Stretches
to firm up the left side of your face

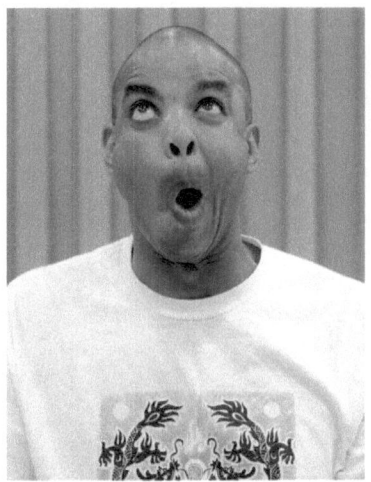

*Figure 31—Starting position for Cheek Stretches
to firm up the right side of your face*

Take your eyebrows and try to make them touch the top of your head. You will feel the skin above your forehead getting tight. Then, squint your face and try to have your eyebrows touch your chin. You will feel the skin above your forehead getting tighter. Do this until your face gets tired. Start slowly, with about 3 sets of 5 repetitions.

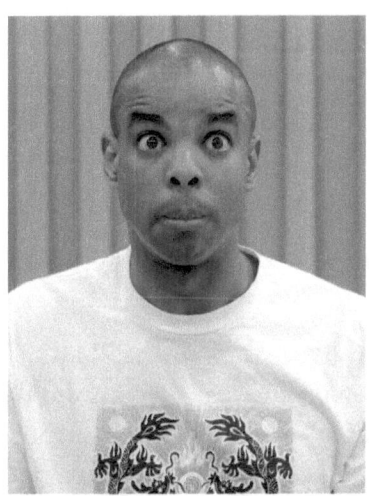

Figure 32—Starting position for Forehead Stretches

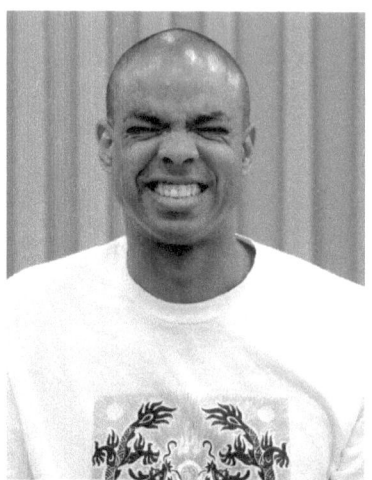

Figure 33—Ending position for Forehead Stretches

Ageless smile

Dentistry has reached a point where you can have minuscule visible signs that you ever had dental work done. Whenever you get any work done on your teeth, always get the work that looks like you didn't have any dental work done in the first place. Very few people, if any, are born with perfect teeth. This only exists as the model for the dental associations. A good cosmetic dentist can get you very close to that model for a price. You may be 50 years old and need braces. Don't hesitate to get them because you think you are too old. You may still live another 70 years looking at your smile. A youthful smile with healthy teeth can boost your self-image and add years to your life.

Remove visible dental work

If you already have visible work, then have it removed as soon as you can afford to. Even if you are not having any dental trouble, if your mouth has visible dental work, go to your dentist and upgrade your smile. Remove all silver and gold fillings in your teeth and replace them with porcelain colors that match the natural color of your teeth. The problem with this advice is your insurance company probably only pays enough to cover 40% to 70% of the standard (and most time cheapest) procedure. The difference will come out of your pocket, but this is money well spent.

The results of this work on your personal self-image will astound you. People will say you look years younger but they can't figure out why. Also, every time you open your mouth to brush your teeth, you see a white, healthy, and beautiful smile. There is no silver, gold, or wire and it feels terrific.

Bleach Your Teeth Every 7 Years

Years of wear and tear and eating certain foods cause your teeth to stain and look dingy. Every seven years get your teeth bleached. You bleach your clothes when they get stains so you can also have your dentist bleach your teeth. No matter how well you brush your teeth, floss, and get regular checkups, your teeth will still be stained. Brushing can only do so much and you need professional bleaching to get out the deep stains that penetrate the enamel.

Ageless eyes

Eyes look older that are bloodshot or dingy in the part that is supposed to be white. The bloodshot look is caused by irritated blood vessels. If your eyes are continually bloodshot, visit your doctor to determine the cause. Also if the white part is dingy, this is cause for concern and you must visit your optician as soon as possible.

Bags Underneath the Eyes

Bags underneath the eyes make you look older. Some people's bags are so big that they begin to look like bruises underneath the eyes. This problem can be hereditary or may result from aging. Eyelid surgery, or blepharoplasty, is needed to remove the excess skin. Exercising the face muscles cannot remove the bags. Covering the bags with make-up sometimes draws more attention to the problem.

Remove crow's feet

Crow's feet are nothing more than wrinkles that appear in the outer corner of your eyes. They are caused by wear and tear on your face, squinting, and smoking. The shape of some people's face makes them more likely to get crow's feet for no reason whatsoever. Depending on the severity of your crow's feet, this is an area where surgery has such outstanding results it is the best option.

The second alternative is to use a cream like retin-a, which has a skin tightening effect. This is a very temporary fix and the effects last only for a few hours.

The final alternative is to cover them with make-up. This is your last alternative for two reasons. First, this alternative is only useful for women, since most men don't wear facial makeup on a regular basis. Secondly, if crow's feet are deep, it may require too much make-up to cover them.

Replace glasses with contact lenses

Wearing glasses makes you appear older looking for several reasons. First, it detracts from your natural face. Second, we subconsciously equate poor vision with older people. Third, wearing glasses causes friction marks on parts of the nose bridge and the back of the ears where the glasses touch the face. Contact lenses correct your vision without making you appear older looking.

The exception to not wearing glasses is on sunny or bright light days when you need to wear sunglasses. Sunglasses protect your eyes by filtering the light to reduce brightness and prevent ultraviolet (UV) and infrared (IR) radiation damage. Wear sunglasses that block at least 95% of the UV and IR radiation. Make sure the protection wraps around the entire eye.

With advances in optical technology you may one day get your eyes tuned up to perfect vision by placing your face into a machine, having a laser beam analyze your eyes and reshape any abnormalities instantly. Presently, don't consider surgical options for at least another ten years. Although corrective eye surgery has been proven safe and thousands of people are doing it, please wait. Remember silicon breast implants?

The benefits of not having to clean contacts have not yet outranked the unknown risks of long-term surgical complications.

Ageless skin

Your skin is the most visible organ of your body. Nothing you can do to any other part of your body provides you with the greatest payback for effort than keeping your skin looking healthy and youthfully taut. In many ways the quality of your skin is analogous to the rings on the tree. The older a tree gets the more rings can be found in the wood grain. Likewise, the older you become the more age related damage is usually found on your skin. Amazingly, your skin constantly replaces itself with new cells daily. Thus, the skin cells that you have at age fifty are not 50-year-old skin cells; they are one-year-old skin cells, residing on a body that has lived 50 years. You might then ask, "Why doesn't the skin look fresh and new when it replaces itself with new skin cells? How come the skin that is replaced looks aged?" The reason for this phenomenon is that your skin cells have a memory. This memory that resides in each cell was aged. Change the memory and you change the cell. In the sections which follow you will learn how to change the memory so that your regenerated skin cells appear as young as you think you are.

How to wash your skin

The three things that make skin look healthy are moisture, tightness and even tone. Moisture happens internally and externally. Internally your cells are well nourished by drinking large amounts of water and eating a balanced healthy diet. Externally moisture is applied using the appropriate creams and oils for your skin type (i.e. dry, normal, or oily). Tightness of skin is accomplished by proper exercise and weight lifting, which is covered extensively in other sections.

Evenness of tone is by far the most important factor from an observational viewpoint. It is the ability to keep your skin the same color; texture and shade that makes you appear young. How you wash your skin and what you use to wash it has a profound impact on the even tone. Consider washing your skin daily with a coca-butter based soap product applied with a washcloth or abrasive pad. Coca butter has the property of blending your skin into an even tone. Just like rubbing compound smoothes out blotches on your car's paint job, coca-butter evens out the blotches and color differences in your skin. It blends away small scars and gives your skin an even tone. You need to apply it to your whole body with a washcloth daily, using the abrasive power of the washcloth to remove dead skin cells. Washing your entire body this way is what gives your body one even tone and makes you appear younger looking.

How to repair sun damaged skin and still have fun

Remember how your new car looked all shiny and bright? Remember how the sun made your car's shiny new paint job faded and dull. Sun damage is also the reason for your skin's weathered appearance. This section provides the steps you must do to repair sun-damaged skin.

Sunshine when used properly is good for you and necessary for the production of vitamin D. But when over-used and abused it damages your skin. Modern culture has leaned toward over exposure. The reason for the over exposure is that suntans give your skin the appearance of an even tone. Regrettably, the sun also robs your skin of its youth due to oxidation, and gives your skin the look of worn leather. Suntans rob moisture from the fat lining underneath your skin and cause premature wrinkles.

Too much sun can cause you to die decades before your time from skin cancer. We have all heard the phrase, "she has a tan to die for." Let's not take this phrase to a literal extreme. If you are very fair skinned and if you live in a warm sunny climate, consider moving. If moving is not possible, then consider wearing clothing that covers your skin. Carrying an oversized umbrella to block the sunrays is also a good idea.

Sun blocks do work, but may provide a false sense of security, which causes you to damage 99 percent of your skin while you protect less than 1 percent--and usually this is your nose and certain parts of your face. Of course, use the sun block for your face; but also wear a hat that covers your neck or carry an umbrella to shield yourself from the sun's rays.

The best sun block is to cover your skin with a layer of white cotton. White cotton is best since it reflects the sun, whereas a dark color absorbs the sun. Cotton is light and breathable so you are also comfortable even in the heat of the sun. Cotton provides a layer of cloth between the sun and your skin, which is the best sun block factor you can buy for your money.

Once you have eliminated over exposure by avoiding direct contact with the sun, then start washing your skin with coca butter based soap, using a washcloth or an abrasive pad to remove the outer layers of your skin that are dry and leathery due to sun damage. Drink plenty of water to not only flush your system of toxic waste, but to also provide nourishment for the fat cells underneath your skin.

This process may take from two to four years before you see the results. But the results are remarkable and well worth the hard work. A person who was 60 with sun-damaged skin can get the skin back to the appearance of a person in their late 30's. This difference is well worth the years of hard work. People want immediate results; otherwise they think it doesn't work. There are no quick solutions to repair sun-damaged skin. It took 20 to 40 years of sun abuse to get the skin in such bad shape. Two to four years is not too long to wait for results that may potentially reverse 20 to 40 years off your appearance and add years to your life.

Lift weights to eliminate most wrinkles

Of all the skin problems that are associated with the aging process, wrinkles truly are a product of growing older. Many of the other problems with your skin are caused by external damage or bad habits, but wrinkles occur naturally as you age. Wrinkles are the result of the lower lining of your skin (which is composed of fat cells) gradually becoming thinner. This causes the upper portion of your skin to sag down into the void that was once supported by the fat layer.

Although wrinkles are natural they are easily controlled. To control the appearance of wrinkles you must become a weight lifter with a goal to produce muscle mass. Weight lifting removes wrinkles by replacing the thinning fat layer with increased muscle mass. Weight lifting can remove wrinkles from 80 percent of your body. The remaining 20 percent are your hands, feet, neck and face, from which wrinkles cannot be removed by lifting weights. The muscles in these areas are very small and do not spread out far enough or increase in mass large enough to replace the thinning fat layer of your skin. In the next section of this chapter, you learn ways to control the wrinkles in these areas. For now the focus is on the 80 percent that weight lifting can correct.

Removing wrinkles or preventing them from appearing on your body takes a lot of hard work at the gym. Some people do not associate lifting weights with wrinkle removal, but for the 80 percent of your body that has the large muscle mass, it is the best method and really the only method worth discussing. Lifting weights to remove wrinkles takes several years to accomplish the desired result, but the rewards are well worth the price. You will only pay the price in time and effort if you really believe that you will get the desired result.

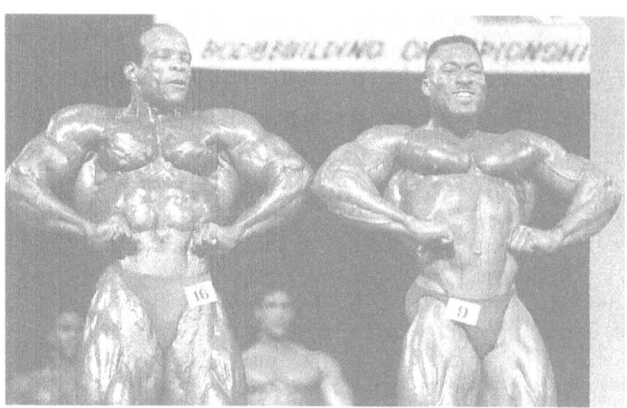

Figure 34—Albert Beckles winning the 1991
Niagara Falls Pro invitational at age 60

To convince yourself to the effectiveness of lifting weights, take a look at the picture of Albert Beckles (on the left) winning the Niagara Falls Pro Invitational only 2 1/2 months from his 61st birthday. At an age when many people are ready to receive social security checks, this man is still competing for the Mr. Olympia contest and placing in the money against people three times younger. You don't have to lift weights and grow muscles big enough to win Mr. Olympia, but you do need them large enough to tighten the skin and fill out the wrinkles. These results work equally for women as they do for men.

There is no excuse to have wrinkles on the 80 percent of your body that has large muscle mass like your arms chest, legs, and torso. We have just accepted as a society that wrinkles are natural and normal (which they are) so let them come as they may. This is the wrong attitude. Start thinking of wrinkles as an indicator that you need to start lifting weights.

Shave all body hair except on the head and eyes

You are about to receive a big secret for an ageless appearance used by fashion models, so remember this one: remove all body hair except your eyebrows, eyelashes, eyelids, and the hair on your head. Furthermore, keep your eyebrows, eyelashes, and eyelids well groomed. All other hair makes you look older than you really are.

Poorly groomed body hair makes you look older and makes everyone else think you are older. The reason the lack of body hair makes you appear younger is that it allows the skin to maintain the appearance of an even tone. Whereas, body hair reflects the light on your body at different angles making your skin appear less even in tone. Many models have no body hair when taking photos since the light reflects off the hair and makes the skin look uneven.

Learn how to shave correctly

Shaving facial hair for men and legs and armpits for women is an accepted grooming norm. Yet for all the shaving that goes on in the world, have you ever heard of a book or video that teaches you how to shave? For many people shaving is one of those chores like taking out the trash--it is not very enjoyable, but a necessary evil. Many people shave so poorly that it causes the opposite effect for which it was done. People shave to appear younger looking, but incorrect shaving ages your skin and your appearance. The following steps describe how to correctly shave your skin:

1. Get in the shower with the water as warm as you can bear.

2. Scrub the skin to be shaved with an abrasive pad covered with coca butter soap.
3. Apply a paste of baking soda to the soap and let it sit for about 2 minutes.
4. Rinse off the area and let the hair absorb the water.
5. Move away from the water and apply shaving cream.
6. Shave one stroke at a time and rinse the razor often.
7. Shave with the pattern and direction of the hair growth.
8. When finished shaving step back into the running water and rinse off.
9. Stay in the shower and drip dry.
10. While the skin is still moist apply Coca-butter lotion or body oil to your entire body.
11. Do this everyday, even when you don't see significant hair growth.

Remove moles

Moles are skin growths that occur on your body for many reasons—some you are born with, while others appear over time. The illusion of youthful skin is an even tone and moles distract from that illusion. The more moles you have, the older you are perceived to be. Remove all moles that your dermatologist says can be safely removed.

This is one area where surgery is the only alternative. There really is no exercise method to remove moles. Improving your diet, exercising, or even applying external creams cannot remove a mole. Depending on where the moles exist, they may be hard to cover up with makeup.

Furthermore, some moles can be potential problems to your health. Certain types of moles can change shape or color and become cancerous. By removing the mole you remove that problem. It is analogous to a car with a little rust spot. Ignored, that little rust spot may not amount to any significant damage, but in certain climates, such as salt-water climates, a little rust spot grows and eventually rusts away the entire car. It is better to just remove the little spot before it becomes a potentially large problem.

The technology to remove moles leaves a small surgical scar that results in an improvement over the original mole. After washing your skin with the coca butter based soap and lotion products, in time that little scar will blend and give your skin an even tone.

Remove age or liver spots

Age or liver spots have nothing to do with your age or liver. These flat dark brown spots are largely the product of years of sun damage. There are many myths about these spots. Some people think these spots occur because their cells can no longer excrete waste properly. Others think it's because their liver is not working as effectively as they age. Many people think that they are permanent because they are flat on the skin.

You might begin seeing these spots in your late 40s to early 50's and they can be removed easily by electro-surgery. There are some chemical applications to remove the spots but many times the chemical side effects can cause problems with the surrounding healthy skin. Once you get rid of these age spots, your behavior that put them there in the first place must change. Protect your skin from the sun by covering up with proper clothing to keep from getting any more.

Remove varicose veins

Varicose veins alter the appearance of an even skin tone because of discoloration. Many times the veins appear blue or green depending on your skin color. Like many of the age indicators, varicose veins have nothing do with the aging process, but more to do with your hormonal process and exercise habits. Varicose veins are rare in men but are very common in women usually after childbirth. Regrettably, there is no exercise to remove varicose veins. Exercise only works to avoid getting them. Avoiding varicose veins involves exercise such as daily walks, tennis and weight lifting for the legs. Also, don't sit in one position for long periods of time. If you do have varicose veins, electro-surgery is the best method to remove them.

Prevent clothing damage to your skin

Clothing masks certain parts of your body from the light, thereby causing uneven tone. Furthermore, clothes or accessories may cause friction marks on parts of your body. You will have friction marks all over your body based on how you wear your clothing. To reduce the damage clothing does to your skin, you must examine your body for friction spots. Since we cannot all become nudists the answer is to eliminate the friction areas as much as possible and to alternate the friction if elimination is impractical. Then use the washcloth and coca butter based soap to help blend the skin tone around the areas that are getting the friction. The majority of friction marks are around the neck (collar rub), around the waist (belt rub), around the breast (bra rub), around the crotch (underwear rub), under the arms (under garment rub) and around the feet and toes (shoe rub).

Ageless hair

The hair on your head is a very noticeable indicator of the aging process. It is easily altered to make you appear younger.

Color your hair if gray

A head full of gray hair is associated with old age and wisdom, but both associations have little basis of truth. Gray hair has little to do with age and there are many people with gray hair that are anything but wise. Gray hair is caused by the under production of melanin. Melanin is the chemical in the blood that provides the colors in your body. When the hormonal production of melanin decreases it causes the hair to receive less and turn gray. The reason for the under production is hormonal and not age related. Gray hair occurs at different times for different people.

Use a hair color you can apply like a shampoo and make coloring a grooming habit as natural as brushing your teeth. Not that you must color out the gray everyday. Do this on a regular basis such as once a week or more depending on your rate of hair growth.

Trim hair that grows where it shouldn't

Let's talk about what to do with hair that is growing wild inside your ears, nose, and on your eyebrows. These are definite signs of aging that make you seem older. Buy yourself a pair of small scissors or have your barber or beautician groom this hair on a regular basis.

Eyebrow hair is another subtle indicator of age. This is hair that many people never groom. It just grows wild and gives you "Albert Einstein" looking eyebrows. The way to eliminate this look is to push against the eyebrows from the ears to the middle of the forehead. This causes all the hair to stand up. Then trim those hairs that have grown too long.

Transplant Hair if Bald

Baldness is another hormonal issue that is not age related. A person with a bald head or thinning hair just naturally looks older than a person with a full head of hair. The best option for baldness is a surgical hair transplant. Hair follicles (plugs) from areas that are not bald are surgically transplanted into identical plugs in the balding area. After the surgery, the hair in the transplanted plug falls out and a scab forms. Within a few weeks the scab heals and new hair begins to grow. This process takes several weeks to complete, but when done right, gives you the best option of all, your own growing hair. This option is expensive, depending on the severity of your baldness. It is money well spent. A full head of hair can take 20 years off your appearance and boost your self-esteem.

Wear a contemporary hair style

In our society there are three styles of hair, contemporary, traditional, and radical. To appear ageless, change with the times and keep your hairstyle contemporary. If you are not sure which hairstyles are contemporary, then subscribe to a magazine such as Vogue for women and GQ for men and look at the hairstyles that best reflect the age you want to project. Also, ask your barber or beautician to keep your style contemporary.

Ageless extremeties

Have you ever seen a person with a regular exercise program for his neck, fingers, or toes? Probably not, and yet these areas make you look years older than necessary, primarily due to a lack of attention. Just imagine how your smile would look if you never brushed your teeth? Likewise, many people never work on these parts of their body as a part of keeping up their appearance. Then they wonder why after 30 to 50 years of neglect, these parts look so much older than the rest of their body.

We live in a world that worships the visible parts. Look around you and you see this worship in everything. Go to your local car wash and notice the people washing and scrubbing their cars, because everyone sees the outside. At jobs people want the most visible assignments because they lead to promotions and praise. People take excellent care of their yards and the exteriors of their houses because that is what everyone can see. Sometimes this "worship of the visible" mentality comes at the expense of neglecting the less visible parts. Many of those less visible parts are the very supports that make the visible possible. For example, neglect the care and maintenance of the engine and that nice shiny car just sits on the side of the road for a tow. Neglect calking your bathroom, or keeping up the heating and plumbing systems and that beautiful looking house will be a very uncomfortable place to live. Neglect the little things on your job and you are soon unemployed. It is the same with your body. The feet, hands, and neck are often neglected because they are deemed not as important as many of the more visible parts of your anatomy.

Give feet the same attention you give hands

Your feet are very important body parts; yet they are the "Rodney Dangerfields" of your anatomy--they get no respect. They provide a very important function for you in providing the ability to stand and to walk. When is the last time you heard someone say they were going to take care of their feet? A good illustration of this point is found in the beauty cream industry. Next time you shop, take note of the product names. You will see many lotions called hand cream, or hand and body lotion. See if you can find one product called foot cream or foot and body lotion. Here we see society implicitly setting subtle rules that imply that foot care and appearance is not important.

Your self-image influences the rate at which your body ages. Based on your mind's belief, you either age quickly or slowly. Since feet are covered up for much of the day you may think, "what the heck, nobody's ever going to see these feet anyway." The problem is you will see them. If they are unsightly, crusty, smelly, blistered, and hairy; you might age 10 years instantly. Feet are your hidden indicator of age; they have a subtle influence on your psyche. How can you feel good about having a face that looks 20 years younger than your real age and then look down at the ground and see feet that look 20 years older than your age? You just can't do it.

The best treatment for old looking feet is exercise. Create an exercise program for your feet, which includes toe raisers, and feet curls. These exercises are important because your feet are covered with very little fat and very little muscle. The top part of the foot is mostly bone, and veins. As long as you keep up the muscle strength, your feet will not wrinkle that much as you age.

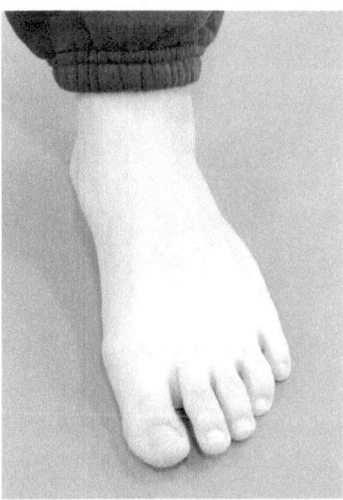

Figure 35—Foot in normal resting position

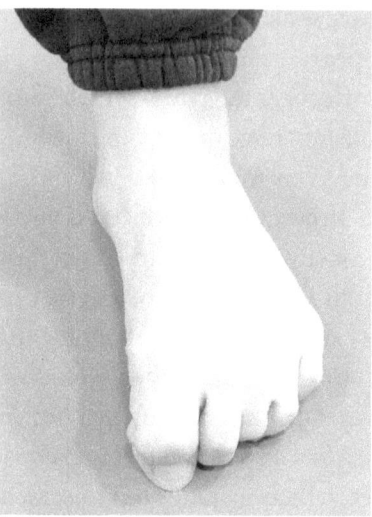

Figure 36—Foot in flexed position

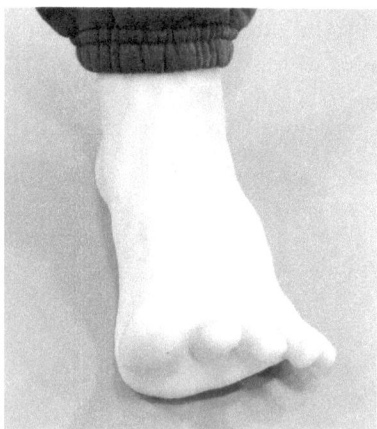

Figure 37—Foot in compressed position

The next step is the proper grooming of your feet. Shave off any hair growing on your feet and toes. Go to the pedicurist as regularly as you go to the barber or hair stylist. Make sure that you get a footbath, callous scrub, and foot massage as part of the process. Keep your feet moisturized with a good foot lotion.

Invest as much money you can afford in high quality leather shoes. Do not buy or wear cheap or tight shoes that cause your feet to have blisters, corns, or calluses. Wear clean socks or stockings everyday. When you are at home wear sandals or any type of shoe that protects the bottom of your feet but does not cover the top. This gives your feet a chance to breathe and soak up natural light.

Wear gloves to protect hands when working

Your hands are one of the hardest working parts of your body. They are also probably the second most neglected body part after the feet. Feet are easier to neglect because they are covered up. Conversely, hands are very visible but are not taken seriously. When is the last time you ever saw or heard of someone doing exercises for their hands?

Your hands can look just as young as the rest of your body. The hands, like the feet, can be kept very healthy looking up to a point. Like the feet, the top and very visible part of the hand (i.e. the backside of your palm) is mostly bone and veins with muscle between the bones. There is very little fat layer, so as the fat layer decreases the wrinkles will not be that deep. The muscle layer is not big enough to fully compensate for the loss of fat. But there is enough muscle to reduce the amount of wrinkles and keep the skin relatively tight.

There are many beneficial exercises for your hands. Fingertip pushups will strengthen the hands and fingers. Doing wrist curls with a small set of dumbbells is a good exercise for the hands. Squeezing a rubber ball or a tennis ball every other day for 100 times is a good exercise for the back of the hands and the palms. This keeps your skin firm and the muscles strong.

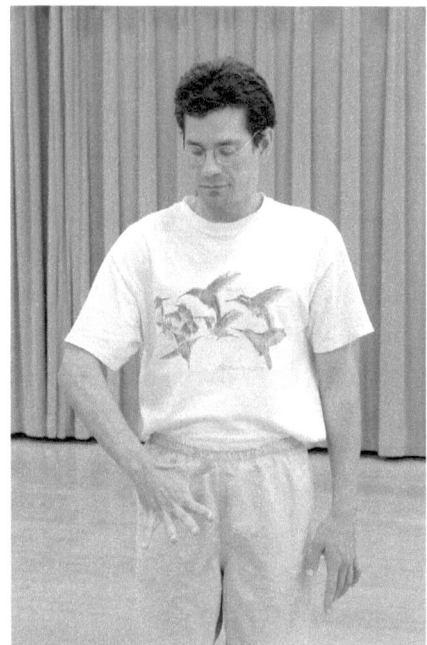

Figure 38—Hands Flexed Exercise

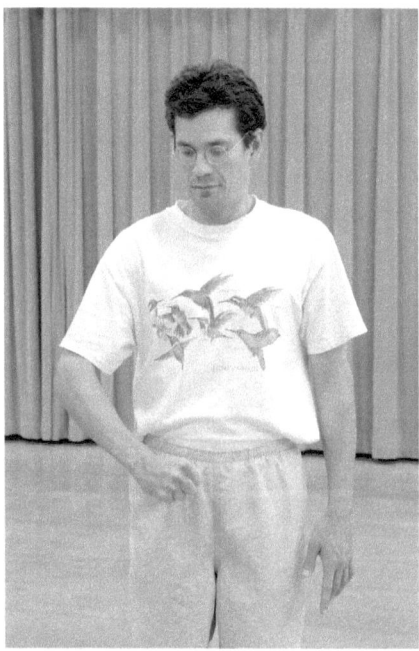

Figure 39—Hands Compressed Exercise

You must cover-up your hands when doing physical labor. Wear gloves for most work activities where you use your hands. Again, this is an area where hands got no respect. Auto mechanics use their hands every day and subject them to cuts, grease, chemical stains, and plenty of hard-core friction and abuse. Yet, have you ever seen an auto mechanic that did his or her job wearing gloves? People take their hands for granted. Protect your hands from the abuse of chemicals and friction in all your work. Wear gloves, whether doing dishes at home or garden work around the house. Any type of work that requires you to use your hands and exposes them to different chemicals or friction also requires gloves to place a layer of protection against the wear and tear.

Finally, clip your nails and visit the manicurist to keep your hands looking good. Trim your nails weekly to promote new nail growth. Untrimmed nails begin to look yellowish. As you age nail growth slows. Cut your nails and file them to stimulate new growth. Keep the hair off the hands and fingers and use hand cream daily. Doing this keeps the hands moist.

Do exercises for your neck and chin

The neck is one body part that never has to look old. Yet, a lot of people rarely if ever exercise their necks. Your neck is a very visible part of the body. Yet, the neck is the twin sister to the feet in getting no respect. The neck needs exercise. Weight lifting and resistance exercises for the neck can replace wrinkles and sagging skin with firm muscles.

Bulky neck muscles have turned many people off to exercising the neck. Some people think that a muscular neck looks unfeminine on a woman and unattractive on a man. For these reasons it is not popular to exercise the neck. The unpopularity of exercising the neck is the leading reason why necks look older than they have too. Granted, big neck muscles might not be that sexy, but we have gone to the other extreme and don't exercise a very important muscle at all.

Eliminate sagging or double chin

A sagging chin or double chin is nothing more than the same wrinkle you see in your neck extending up the bottom of your chin.

Take a moment to touch your neck and feel the muscles that are in it. There are some that go up the back of the head, and some that go up under the chin. Keep the muscles in the neck firm and tight to eliminate that double or triple chin look.

Exercises to remove wrinkles from the neck and chin

Here are several exercises you can do to remove any wrinkles in your neck and keep it looking ageless. The first few exercises are resistance exercises and you will need a partner. Get on your hands and knees and turn your neck so it is looking up at the ceiling. Your partner stands in front of you and place his or her hands under your chin. Then with all your might pull your neck down till it touches your chest. Your partner applies resistance, so that the process takes 10 seconds. Start with 3 sets of 5 repetitions each. This exercise firms up the skin under your chin as well as the front muscles of your neck. This skin becomes firm because the muscles in the neck expands and absorb the excess wrinkled skin from the chin area.

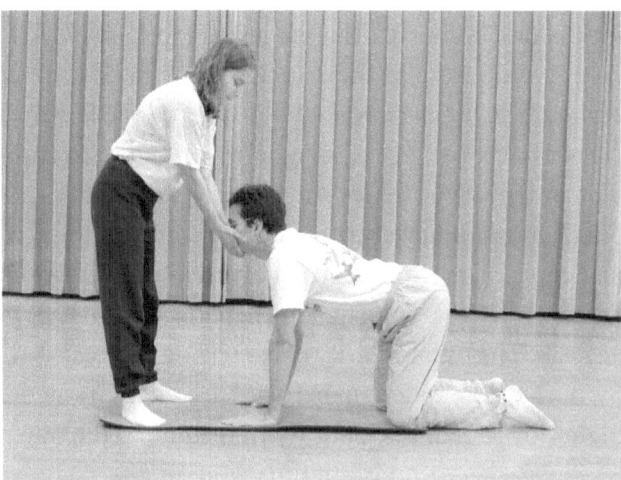

Figure 40—Starting position for front of neck and chin exercise

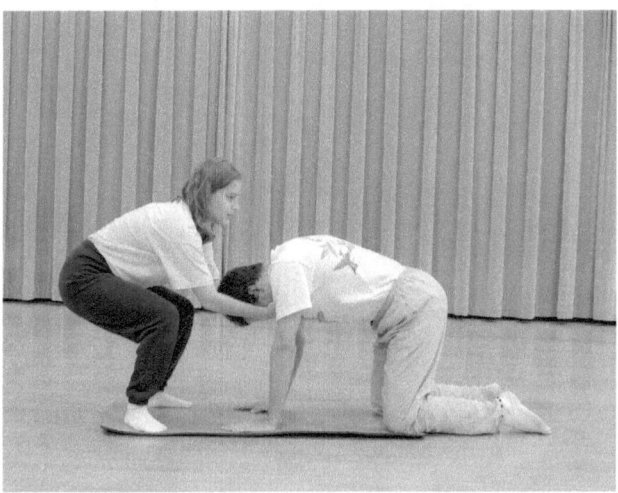

Figure 41—Ending position for front of neck and chin exercise

The next resistance exercise is to move the neck in the opposite direction. Place your chin on your chest. Your partner then provides resistance to the back of your head. Your objective is to move your neck so that you are looking up at the ceiling. Your partner applies resistance, so that the process takes 10 seconds. Start with 3 sets of 5 repetitions each. This exercise firms up the skin on the back of your neck.

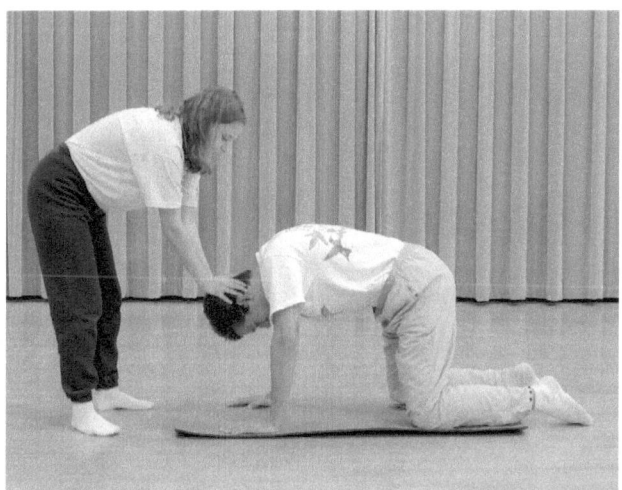

Figure 42—Starting position for back of neck and chin exercise

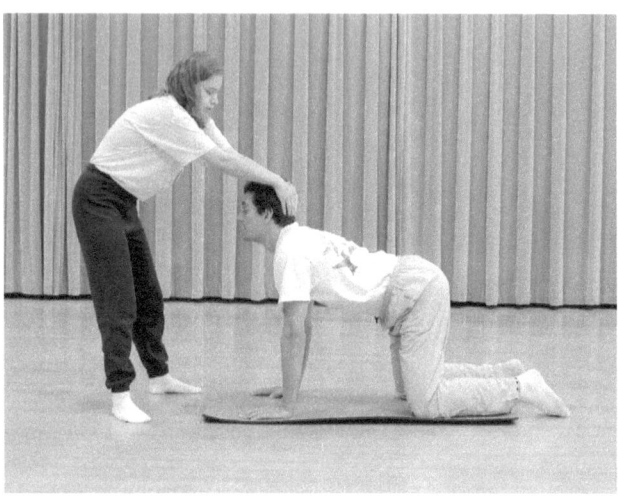

Figure 43—Ending position for back of neck and chin exercise

The next resistance exercise is to move the neck from the right to the left. Place your right ear on your right shoulder. Your partner then provides resistance to the left side of your head. Your objective is to move your neck so that your left ear touches your left shoulder. Your partner applies resistance, so that the process takes 10 seconds. Start with 3 sets of 5 repetitions each. This exercise firms up the muscles on the left side of your neck.

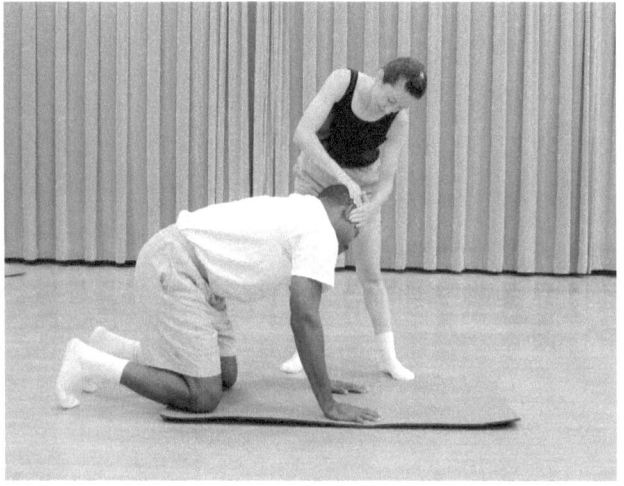

Figure 44—Starting position for side of neck exercise

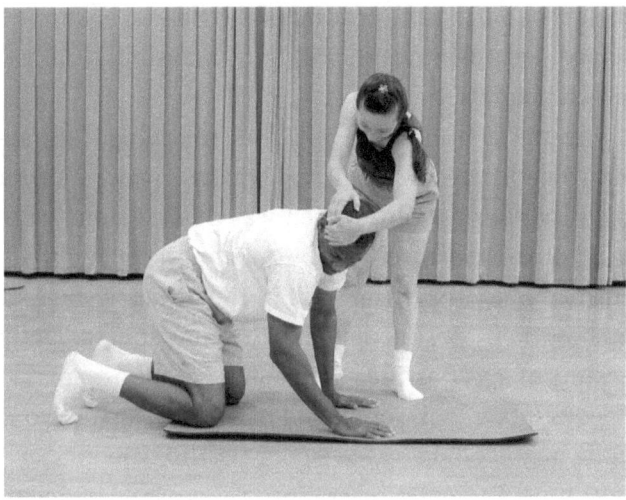

Figure 45—Ending position for side of neck exercise

Your final resistance exercise is to move the neck from the left to the right. Place your left ear on your left shoulder. Your partner then provides resistance to the right side of your head. Your objective is to move your neck so that your right ear touches your right shoulder. Your partner applies resistance, so that the process takes 10 seconds. Start with 3 sets of 5 repetitions each. This exercise firms up the muscles on the right side of your neck.

There are several weight lifting machines that provide the same neck resistance movement just described. Check with your health club. If the club has the machines, then repeat the exercises using weights. Again, your objective is to replace the decreasing fat with increasing muscle, to eliminate any wrinkles that can occur. Since you have never exercised these muscles before, expect some soreness. Don't let this pain scare you away from continuing your exercise program. Any muscle that has never been exercised will have pain in the beginning. Finally, before beginning any neck exercise program please consult your doctor or chiropractor first.

Ageless posture

A person's posture is a visible indicator of age. When you think of a very old person you visualize them as stooped over with a hump back and head held low. This is the posture of the elderly, or so you think. In reality, this old age posture is the result of many years of bad posture habits of youth magnified.

When you think of youth, you think of strong, tall, and sturdy posture with head held high. In reality, the majority of our young people have very poor posture. When was the last time you were ever instructed on proper posture? Maybe your mother taught you how to walk for the big dance, or if you were in the military you had to learn to stand at attention. Most people like to stand at ease. Unlike all the other indicators of age, posture cannot stand alone and make you look old. This means if you look young and have poor posture you still look young, but if you look old and have poor posture you look even older.

Good posture eliminates several problems associated with old age; one being lower back pain and the other being a humped back (i.e. Kyphosis or Hyperlordosis). When your posture is not correct, your body has to compensate for the alignment problem by either stretching the muscles or bones. This principle of alignment and structural stress is important to the profession of chiropractors and structural engineers. Your body is a structure, subject to stresses when things are not in proper alignment. When your neck is not in its proper position the muscles have to over compensate. This may not be a problem in your youth, but as you become older this overcompensation is unnecessary work. Many times your body switches rather than fights and provides bone growth to compensate for years of bad habits. The curved spine is an effect of a bad posture habit and not enough dietary calcium in the bones over a lifetime. This is not a cause of old age; it is an effect of poor habits. In life you reap what you sow. Start the habit of good posture and proper calcium in your diet and many of the stresses of improper body alignment may not occur in your body.

Learn how to know if your posture is correct

Having proper knowledge of what good posture looks like and how to achieve it is the best way to improve your posture. Proper posture is necessary for long life. What does proper posture feel like and look like? Proper posture can be learned but you have to use it when you are young (before age 40) to get the best results. Otherwise, your muscles may not be able to properly do the work. Do not allow the buttocks to protrude or the back to swoop inward in swayback fashion.

Find a wall and put your back to the wall, then make sure your heels, buttocks, shoulder blades, and the back of your head touche the wall. Your eyes and chin are parallel to the floor (i.e. look straight ahead). This is good posture. If it feels strange to you then you probably have poor posture.

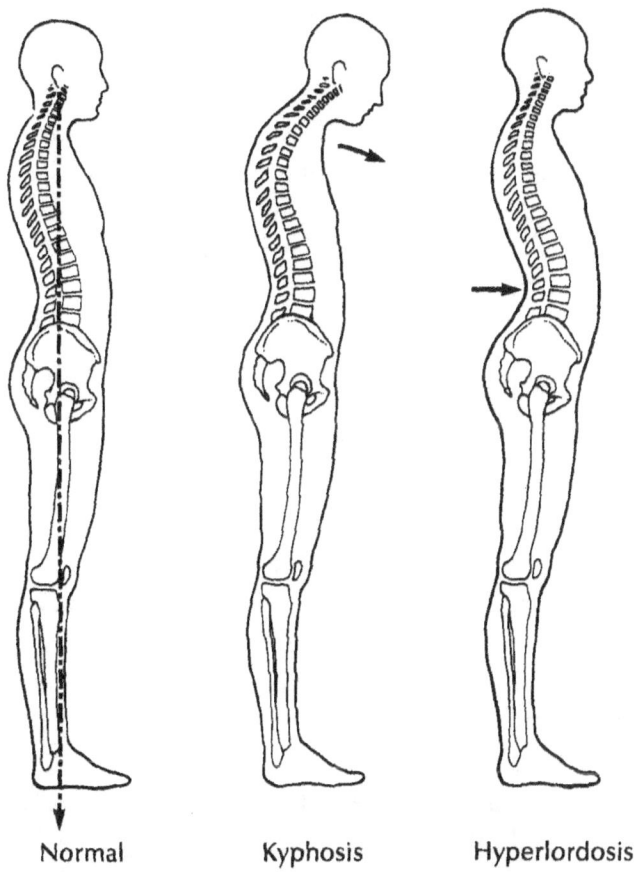

Normal   Kyphosis   Hyperlordosis

*Figure 46—Illustration from the Columbia
University Complete Home Medical Guide*

Breathe deeply and slowly

Proper posture also provides you the benefit of deeper breathing. Over the course of a lifetime deeper breathing adds years to your life span because your body is getting the necessary air it needs to survive. Some of the headaches that you experience are due to the body not getting the adequate amounts of air. That pain is a message to breathe deeper. Improper posture inhibits your ability to breathe deeply and fill your body with fresh air with every breath.

To illustrate the effects of poor posture on your ability to breathe, find a chair that has a backrest and bend your back and try to place your head between your knees. In this position breathe as deeply as possible. You will notice that you cannot fill your lungs unless you straighten up your back. This exercise illustrates the worst posture possible for breathing. Yet, many people are so stooped over as a result of poor posture that this exaggerated poor-posture exercise is not far from the reality of their breathing.

Ageless voice

An auditory indicator of age is your voice. Ever receive a call from a stranger? Just from the sound of his or her voice you have a very clear idea of the person's stage in life. You can immediately tell if an adolescent answers the telephone, a child, a teenager or an elderly person. But it is difficult to determine an adult's age (i.e. from 25 to 65 years of age) just by the sound of the voice. After 65, the voice starts to get more graveled in sound due to larger build up of mucus in the larynx and decreased muscle flexibility of the vocal cords. Although it is difficult to determine a person's exact age from their voice, it is very easy to see the difference between a 25 year old and a 65 year old in appearance. This is why your voice is a truer reflection of who you are and how you really age. It is part of that invisible realm of life that is divine, eternal and pure energy.

If you have the voice of an old person, you subconsciously appear old to the listener every time you open your mouth. No matter how young you look, if you sound old, people see you as old. Remember Spanky from the "Little Rascals?" He was a little kid, but everyone saw him as an old man because he had an old man's voice.

The good news is your voice need not sound old until you are well over 100 years old. You can easily have the same voice you have in your 20's well into the century mark of your life. You will now learn how to keep your voice sounding youthfully vibrant all throughout your life. Keeping your voice youthfully vibrant requires just four things: drink plenty of water, sing every day, exercise your neck, and don't smoke anything.

Drink plenty of water

You already know the benefits drinking water has on flushing toxic waste from your body. Another added benefit is water clears out the mucus buildup in your vocal cords and esophagus. As you age, your sinus cavities deteriorate and cause more mucus to enter your throat. This is one of the reasons peoples voices sound deeper and graveled over time. By washing the mucus away your voice does not have to travel through it and sound graveled. Your voice is not graveled, it just has to travel though mucous. The water clears away this obstacle.

Sing every day

We live in a universe. Uni means one, and verse means song--thank you Alan Watts. Thus, the word universe can be translated into the phrase "one song." When you sing you are connecting that spiritual dimension of your voice with its true nature, the universe. Singing places your soul in another dimension. Have your ever seen a person singing that was not truly happy? I don't mean one who is performing for pay as a job, but a person just walking down the street with a song in their heart and voice. Usually, people only sing when they are happy. Sing and it makes you happy.

Singing also provides the exercise for your vocal cords that is necessary to keep your voice youthful. Just like a musical instrument, your voice has a range. When you talk to others, you talk at a certain range. Many people never use the upper and lower limits of their voice. They might exercise the upper limits screaming occasionally when upset, at a sporting event, praising the Lord at worship service, or from pain, but never on a regular basis. If unused, the vocal cords atrophy at those ranges from lack of use. This is why it is important to sing every day.

Exercise your neck

Another reason you voice will sound older is because the neck surrounding the larynx and the vocal cords is never exercised. There are people that have lived 60 or 70 years and never once in their life exercised their neck muscles. The average person never exercises the neck. Then they wonder why they sound so old. Your voice does not age; it is the body around your voice that is aging. Keeping your neck strong prevents the rapid deterioration that claims from some people the voice of their youth.

Don't smoke anything

Smoking destroys the vocal cords and throat. It provides more mucus build up and slowly fries the mouth. Not only does your voice have to travel though the mucus, now it has to travel through the smoke. Please don't smoke.

How old would you be if people guessed your age?

To get an accurate indication of the age people perceive you to be, take random surveys from time to time. Some of the best places to do this are in shopping malls and supermarkets. Please pick people that you think might be older than you. Pick total strangers that have no vested interest in stroking your ego. Politely approach the person and tell them you are doing a survey for research on age perception and you would like them to honestly guess your age. Please ask them not to try to guess higher or lower to be nice or cynical, but to honestly try to guess your age if they had to give your description to the police. They can also give your age in a 3-year range (e.g. 41 to 43). When they give you their guess say thank you and walk away. If they press you to determine if they were right or wrong with their guess politely tell them they were pretty close. Your age is nobody's business.

Perform this exercise on at least 10 different people. If some people gave you a range instead of a specific number, then use the middle number in that range. Take an average of the 10 guesses and you will have a pretty accurate picture of how old you appear to others.

Bibliography for the 6th Principle

1. Age Erasers for Men & Women, Rodale Press
2. American Health for Women, Susan S. Buckley Publisher, 1-800-365-5005
3. Family Circle Magazine, Look Years Younger, 5/13/97 edition
4. Forever Fit: The Lifetime Plan for Health, Fitness, & Beauty, Cher & Robert Haas, Pantam Press
5. How to Wash your Face, Barney J. Kenet MD, Simon & Schuster
6. Learning the Human Game, Alan Watts, Audio Wisdom
7. Muscle & Fitness Magazine, Weider Publications
8. Psycho-Cybernetics, Dr. Maxwell Maltz, Bobbe Sommer, Fine Communications
9. Success and the Self-Image, Zig Ziglar, Simon & Schuster Audio
10. Super Skin: A Leading Dermatologist's Guide to the Latest Breakthrough In Skin Care, Nelson L. Novick, Potter Publishing
11. The Columbia University College Home Medical Guide, Crown Publishing
12. The Road Less Traveled, M. Scott Peck, Simon & Schuster
13. The Thinking Man's Guide to Hair Loss, L. Lee Bosley M.D., The Bosley Medical Institute
14. You Can Heal Yourself, Louise L. Hay, Hay House

EPILOGUE

You have just read a series of practical and workable techniques for living longer, aging slower, and looking younger. You are lucky to be born during the time in history where humans now have the technology and the knowledge to finally live 120 years on average in excellent health as promised by God (Genesis 6:3). Examples have been given of people who have applied the suggested techniques and produced remarkable results. If they can do it, then so can you. But just reading this book is not enough--you must now put to practice what you have just read.

I wrote this book to share with you the six ageless principles for long life success. Again, these principles are:

1. Relax your mind and body with spiritual recreation.
2. Cultivate positive healthy relationships and eliminate the negative.
3. Think and grow healthy, wealthy, and wise.
4. Invest more on yourself than you do on your job and possessions.
5. Exercise before eating and thoroughly flush your system.
6. Refuse to age gracefully.

I have absolute confidence and belief in the methods outlined in this book. Not a day goes by that I am not somehow reminded that these principles are producing dramatic results in my life. By practicing these principles, you too may share in these dramatic results. These principles have been tested in the laboratory of everyday life. They work when worked.

We may never get a chance to meet face to face, but the fact that you have read this books tells me that we are kindred spirits. Therefore, it is my hope that you live long, prosper, and be in good health even as your soul prospers.

Peace & Love,
Andrew Lee Oliver

ABOUT THE AUTHOR

Through this book I wish to share with you some simple discoveries that can produce remarkable results in slowing the aging process. It has worked for me, and for countless others that have either stumbled onto the basics of halting aging, or have just been lucky enough to practice it blindly without knowing it. They, like I, live very rich and fulfilling lives, looking decades younger than they really are, and feeling as young as they look.

My interest in physical fitness began when I set a goal to become an Olympic track competitor. Although I excelled in running and jumping in high school, college, and at some world class meets, I never got over that hurdle to move to the next level. I now realize that, although I had the ability and talent, I was only fooling myself that I was really committed to winning. I was not willing to pay the price to be an Olympian. However, the basis was set for a lifetime of healthful, youthful living, and enjoying other avenues that I would not have considered back in those times. I now teach yoga, meditation and tai chi at Rutgers University. In addition to being a certified black belt in Tae Kwon Do, I am a certified PADI scuba diving instructor; hold masters degrees in computer science, theology, and philosophy. I teach seminars on halting the aging process and I live a rich and fulfilling life. I maintain a healthy, youthful body.

Please observe that I said I maintained a youthful body, and not youthful looking; for that is the crux of this book. I would like to share with you understandable, yet little practiced secrets of living in a manner that allows you to live well over 100 years, and remain in good health until you expire to the next dimension of existence.

Peace & Love,
Andrew Lee Oliver

www.ingramcontent.com/pod-product-compliance
Lightning Source LLC
Chambersburg PA
CBHW061259280526
45784CB00002B/820